To Dear Dr Higgins

Ruth Bull

and

Marie Gelosmeno

HUMANISM IN MEDICINE

ON THE AFTERNOON OF APRIL 22, 1970

Thoughts do live on!
    They can become a way of life,
And all within the work of day:
    Thoughts can live on!
And do, when we remember them
    And pass them on, to others on the way.

How thrilling after more than fifty years
    To listen, in a far off place,
To thoughts so well expressed,
    And always with a smiling face,
By Osler, humanist supreme!
    It is, as Penfield found, a dream.

So, welcome here amongst us, students who
    So greatly carried on
The master's Way of Life!
    Ah! Holman, Penfield, Davison,
And with your wives, you may surmise
    How well you make his thoughts live on, —
A stirring obligato to
    The harmonies that are your own!

Written by Chauncey Leake while listening to Penfield's address

HUMANISM
IN MEDICINE

Edited by

JOHN P. McGOVERN, M.D., Sc.D., LL.D., L.H.D.
Professor and Chairman
Department of History of Medicine
Clinical Professor of Allergy
University of Texas Graduate School of
Biomedical Sciences at Houston
Clinical Professor of
Pediatrics (Allergy) and Microbiology
Baylor College of Medicine
Director
McGovern Allergy Clinic
Houston, Texas

and

CHESTER R. BURNS, M.D., Ph.D.
James Wade Rockwell Assistant Professor of the
History of Medicine
Director of the History of Medicine Division
University of Texas
Medical Branch at Galveston
Galveston, Texas

With a Foreword by
Wilburt C. Davison, M.D., Sc.D., LL.D.
Emeritus Dean
Professor of Pediatrics
Duke University Medical Center
Durham, North Carolina

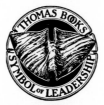

CHARLES C THOMAS • PUBLISHER
Springfield • Illinois • U.S.A.

Published and Distributed Throughout the World by

CHARLES C THOMAS • PUBLISHER

BANNERSTONE HOUSE

301-327 East Lawrence Avenue, Springfield, Illinois, U.S.A.

©1973, by CHARLES C THOMAS • PUBLISHER

ISBN 0-398-02603-3

Library of Congress Catalog Card Number: 72-93222

*With THOMAS BOOKS careful attention is given to all details of
manufacturing and design. It is the Publisher's desire to present books that are
satisfactory as to their physical qualities and artistic possibilities and
appropriate for their particular use. THOMAS BOOKS will be true to those
laws of quality that assure a good name and good will.*

Printed in the United States of America

A-2

Contributors

Donald G. Bates, M.D., *Chairman, Department of the History of Medicine, Faculty of Medicine, McGill University, Montreal, Canada.*

William B. Bean, M.D., *Sir William Osler Professor of Medicine, Department of Internal Medicine, University of Iowa College of Medicine, Iowa City, Iowa.*

Wilburt C. Davison, M.D., *Emeritus Dean and Professor of Pediatrics, Duke University Medical Center, Durham, North Carolina.* (Deceased).

George T. Harrell, M.D., *Dean, Pennsylvania State University College of Medicine and Director, Milton S. Hershey Medical Center, Hershey, Pennsylvania.*

Alfred R. Henderson, M.D., *Consultant, Division of Medical Sciences, Smithsonian Institution, Washington, D.C.*

Hebbel E. Hoff, M.D., Ph.D., *Benjamin F. Hambleton Professor and Chairman of the Department of Physiology, Associate Dean for Faculty and Clinical Affairs, Baylor College of Medicine, Houston, Texas.*

Emile Holman, M.D., *Professor of Surgery Emeritus, Stanford University Medical School, Stanford, California.*

R. Palmer Howard, M.D., *Professor of the History of Medicine, University of Oklahoma Medical Center, Oklahoma City, Oklahoma.*

Lester S. King, M.D., *Senior Editor,* Journal of the American Medical Association, *and Professorial Lecturer in the History of Medicine, University of Chicago, Chicago, Illinois.*

James A. Knight, M.D., *Associate Dean and Professor of Psychiatry, Tulane University School of Medicine, New Orleans, Louisiana.*

Wilder G. Penfield, M.D., *Honorary Consultant, Montreal Neurological Institute and Hospital, Montreal, Canada.*

Charles G. Roland, M.D., *Chairman, Department of the Medical Library and of Publications, Mayo Foundation, Rochester, Minnesota.*

H. Grant Taylor, M.D., Dean, *Division of Continuing Education, University of Texas Graduate School of Biomedical Sciences at Houston, Houston, Texas.*

"We are here not to get all we can out of life for ourselves, but to try to make the lives of others happier. It is not possible for anyone to have better opportunities to live this lesson than you will enjoy. The practice of medicine is an art, not a trade; a calling, not a business; a calling in which your heart will be exercised equally with your head."

Osler: The Master Word in Medicine

"In the hospital, we learn to scan gently our brother man, judging not, asking no questions, but meting out to all alike a hospitality worthy of the *Hôtel Dieu,* and deeming ourselves honoured in being allowed to act as its dispensers."

Osler: Doctor & Nurse

"I say advisedly an honest heart—the honest head is prone to be cold and stern, given to judgment, not mercy, and not always willing to entertain that true charity which, while it thinkest no evil, is anxious to put the best possible interpretation upon the motives of a fellow worker. It will foster, too, an attitude of generous, friendly rivalry untinged by the green peril, jealousy, that is the best preventive of the growth of a bastard scientific spirit—loving seclusion and working in a lock-and-key laboratory, as timorous of light as is a thief."

Osler: The Student Life

FOREWORD

As indicated in the following papers, among the many virtues of Sir William Osler was his spontaneous, natural, and kindly interest in patients and students, and in people in general. He practiced this humanism even when his friends were unconsciously rude. For example, at a tea a loud-voiced American woman rudely asked him "Do you prefer being called 'Sir William' or just plain American 'Dr. Osler'?" He smilingly quoted Lewis Carroll's *The Hunting of the Snark*: "I answer to Hi or any loud cry" without hurting her feelings.

WILBURT C. DAVISON

PREFACE

Following the annual meeting of the Association of American Medical Colleges in November of 1968, Dr. John P. McGovern and I agreed to mark the 50th anniversary of the death of Sir William Osler with a symposium. There was such a striking similarity between what the medical students attending the AAMC meeting advocated as desirable modifications in the medical school curriculum and the principles to which Osler dedicated his life's work that several questions came immediately to mind. Do medical students, interns and residents no longer know of Osler and the relevance of his championship of bedside teaching? Are Osler's contributions to preceding generations of medical students no longer applicable? Is Osler's sphere of influence coming to an end? Is the scholarliness and humaneness for which our profession has consistently strived now to be considered non-essential? Will a contemporary Osler emerge or can we make the one we know and love live again?

It seemed to us that the time was optimal to provide some answers to these questions by assembling three distinguished students of Osler and a battery of outstanding speakers to interact in symposium fashion. We also hoped to emphasize a current need for humanism in medicine, to bring Osler to the aid of a troubled profession, and to pay tribute and acknowledge our indebtedness to Sir William. As the scope of this symposium materialized, its substance seemed appropriately circumscribed by the title, "Humanism in Medicine, As Portrayed by the Life of Sir William Osler."

President Truman G. Blocker of the University of Texas Medical Branch at Galveston agreed to sponsor this symposium under the joint auspices of two medical components of The University of Texas System and generously proposed that the program be held at Galveston in the spring of 1970. This was a most fortuitous site and date since our meeting could be scheduled to coincide with the 1970 SAMA-UTMB National Student Research Forum and thereby provide an opportunity for participation by these outstanding student representatives from many American medical schools.

It is our hope that the spirit of Osler, so alive and vibrant at the symposium, can be extended to include the reader through the medium of this monograph and that the reader will conclude with us:

"No one has taken Osler's place. We must demonstrate to this generation not only what he was and meant to us, but what he did for them and for medicine, and can continue to do if the medical youth will try to emulate him as we attempted to do. He embodied, applied, and transmitted all that is finest and best in a physician."*

GRANT TAYLOR

---

*Davison, Wilburt C.: The basis of Sir William Osler's influence in medicine. *Annals of Allergy,* 27:366-372, 1969.

INTRODUCTION

Humanism can denote a special regard for humanistic studies, a pervasive concern for human welfare, or a philosophy that regards natural man as essentially valuable. Since the days of antiquity, man's quest for health has been punctuated with one or more of these expressions of humanism. With today's onrush of scientific and social changes, the spectrum of professional and social values associated with medical education, science, and practice is undergoing widespread, critical review. As one of these review efforts, our symposium posed these questions: What manifestations of humanism can be found in the history of medicine? Why is William Osler revered as a medical humanist? Does humanism have a place in the construction of goals and priorities in medicine? The following essays provide some answers to these questions.

In the first two essays, Lester King and Hebbel Hoff submit strikingly different answers about the manifestations of humanism in the history of medicine. King depicts the impact of Renaissance humanism on the lives of three leading physicians of that era: Linacre, Rabelais, Caius. Hoff is concerned about man's tendency to turn his great men into gods and then to expect these great men to behave like God. With a focus on Paracelsus, Van Helmont, Galvani, Hunter, and the trio involved with ether—Jackson, Morton, Wells—Hoff claims that moral perfection and greatness are not necessarily synonymous. By characterizing some of the eternal ingredients of humanism, King and Hoff set the stage for the remaining essays.

The next eight papers deal with William Osler. The first were written by three eminent Oslerians who actually studied with Sir William at Oxford: Emile Holman, Wilburt Davison, Wilder Penfield. Curiously reinforcing Hoff's assertions, Holman claims that Halsted, with his introversion and addiction, was no less humanistic than Osler with his compassionate friendliness. Davison examines Osler's stated opposition to "full-time" clinical professorships and emphasizes Osler's conviction that clinical medicine cannot be taught effectively by persons who are primarily committed to laboratory investigation. After tracing Osler's humanistic influence upon himself, Penfield, with dramatic skill, re-affirms the everlasting power of Osler's "way of life."

The other five essays offer additional insights into the characteristics of Osler. Palmer Howard discusses the lives of some of the men who directly and indirectly influenced Osler. The irrepressible humor and wit of Osler are depicted in William Bean's analysis of his practical jokes and the E. Y. Davis alias. In contrast, an excerpt from Bean's first presidential address to the

American Osler Society portrays Osler's warm and poignant response to the death of a beloved colleague. By focusing on the qualities of equanimity, detachment, and humanism, Alfred Henderson vividly depicts Osler's abhorrence of war. By examining Osler's travel letters, Charles Roland presents penetrating comments about Osler's humanism, comments that serve as appropriate conclusions for this second portion of the book.

Do Osler and humanism have any meaning for the medical professional of today and tomorrow? With extraordinary perceptiveness, James Knight correlates Osler's philosophy with the needs of today's medical students. The first department of humanities in an American medical school was established at Hershey, Pennsylvania by George Harrell. Harrell reviews the assumptions that undergird this new department and describes some of the efforts to provide a deeper and richer humanistic education for future physicians. In the final paper, Donald Bates circumscribes the attitudes that can serve as specific objectives for those who wish to infuse humanism into medical education. These attitudes include a depth of understanding, the wonders of personal interaction, the security of mutual respect, and the renewal of one's self-understanding—attitudes that can be cultivated by all health professionals.

Not surprisingly, our original questions were not answered completely. Others were raised. When will medical philosophers begin to learn some philosophy? How can ethical problems in medicine be resolved without a better understanding of ethics? What are the relationships or lack thereof between studies in the humanities and the development of humane and humanistic attitudes? Is the future of humanism in medicine a matter of teaching humanities in medical schools or a matter of defining desired attitudes and determining ways to cultivate these attitudes, or both? We hope that other physicians and humanists will respond individually and collectively to these questions.

In publishing the proceedings of our symposium, we have not attempted to mold every paper into a uniform editorial format. In order to retain the individual style, feeling, and humanism that was exhibited during each presentation at the symposium, we have made only minor editorial alterations. We earnestly hope that this volume will not be considered just another eulogy to the great Sir William Osler. For although we wish to bring again to the profession, especially to medical students, the lessons of his life in terms of humanism—it is the potential for humanism in medicine that we wish to emphasize.

The practice of medicine requires knowledge and skill, frequently labeled as the science and art of medicine. Yet, knowledge and skill are incomplete without the directiveness of human goals and objectives. The re-examination of these values in medicine and society will continue as long as physicians and other health professionals strive to understand and renew their ideals.

JOHN P. MCGOVERN AND CHESTER R. BURNS

ACKNOWLEDGMENTS

First, a special note of gratitude is extended to President Truman G. Blocker for the warm and delightful hospitality that he provided for the guest lecturers and their ladies and more personally for his timely comments made throughout the meeting. To members of his faculty who acted as local hosts for our honored guests and their wives, we also offer our thanks.

Many persons made important contributions to the overall success of this symposium. Of special significance were those made by Dr. Robert D. Moreton, Miss Jacqueline McCord, and Mrs. Helen Ayachi.

Never were funds more graciously provided for a symposium. The pharmaceutical industry was particularly enthusiastic, and the following persons deserve special credit: Dr. John B. Jewell, Executive Vice-president and Medical Director, Ayerst Laboratories, New York, New York; Dr. Kenneth G. Kohlstaedt, Vice-president, Medical Research, The Lilly Research Laboratories, Eli Lilly and Company, Indianapolis, Indiana; Mr. R. R. Buntaine, Director of Advertising, Mallinckrodt Pharmaceuticals, St. Louis, Missouri; Dr. Paul A. Walter, Vice-president and Medical Director, Mead-Johnson Research Center, Evansville, Indiana; Dr. Ralph E. Snyder, Director of Professional Relations, Merck Sharp & Dohme, Division of Merck and Company, Inc., Rahway, New Jersey; Dr. B. V. Pisha, Assistant Director, Professional Relations, Roche Laboratories, Division of Hoffmann-La Roche, Inc., Nutley, New Jersey; Dr. Howard W. Baldock, E. R. Squibb and Sons, Inc., New York, New York; Dr. Vincent J. Gagliardi, Medical Director, Regulatory Affairs, Wallace Pharmaceuticals, Cranbury, New Jersey.

Additional support was provided by the University of Texas Medical Branch, the University of Texas Graduate School of Biomedical Sciences at Houston and its Division of Continuing Education, the Texas Allergy Research Foundation, and the McGovern Allergy Clinic.

CONTENTS

Humanism In Medicine

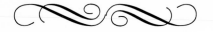

Essay I

Humanism and the Medical Past*

LESTER S. KING, M.D.

THE WORD "HUMANISM" has almost as many meanings as there are people who use it. As a historical term it has many fine shadings, important for understanding the past, while in the present it has distinct meanings in different categories—theology, philosophy, education. And within each of these are further shadings. To discuss humanism in medicine we must limit ourselves sharply.

In the realm of education the humanist would say that our medical teaching lays too much stress on science and not enough on a group of subjects loosely called the humanities. I will not try to define or even enumerate these but they have in common an emphasis on man as a person, as an individual who has ideals and values; who faces conflicts and disappointments; who experiences joys and fulfillment; who lives in a world of qualities and meanings, the rich real world portrayed in novels and poetry and drama and art. All these stand in sharp contrast with the world of quan-

tity and pale abstraction with which science deals. Humanism, emphasizing the world of quality and value, holds that training in these subjects is essential to the physician. Consequently, the humanist would replace much of our "hard" science with something else.

Today we are witnessing a strong trend toward humanism in medicine. An increasing number of critics are insisting that medical students need to be taught a great deal more than the so-called basic sciences and clinical medicine. The physician who intends to provide health care today must know many other things. In recent months, for example, one medical student maintained, "There is an immediate need for the inclusion of sociology, Black history, economics, psychology, and anthropology into the basic science core curricula."[1] A mature leader in medicine declared that physicians must have ". . . knowledge of people, history, social sciences, literature, and art because the doctors must relate the mysteries of the human body to the rest of the society."[2]

These are merely two voices from a growing chorus. We must notice, however, the rather divergent trends in these quotations. On the one hand is a call actually for more science, but in subjects quite different from the physics, chemistry, and biology that make up the underpinning of

*From King, Lester S.: Humanism and the medical past. *JAMA, 213*:580-584, 1970.

medical education. Instead of these "hard" sciences, there is a plea for certain of the "soft" social sciences, particularly sociology, anthropology, and psychology. These, by virtue of their subject matter, do not have the rigor or precision of physics and chemistry but they represent "science" nevertheless. On the other hand, a second trend calls for the humanities in the stricter sense—literature, art, philosophy, and history.

There is much in favor of adding different sciences to those presently taught. Sociology, for example, may be more important than gross anatomy or embryology. The so-called sciences of man might indeed be more significant for the medicine of tomorrow than the sciences currently taught. But the curriculum which contains such new sciences does not thereby become more humanistic, any more than did the curricula in the mid-nineteenth century when courses in physical diagnosis and microscopy were added. The new courses merely reflected the new medical needs, and these projected changes should not be distinguished from the "humanities" in the stricter sense.

Now, in order to pursue this subject, we must go outside the field of medicine and enter a wider cultural area. In the history of culture and the history of ideas the term humanism applies to a movement which reached a climax in the fifteenth and sixteenth centuries. It had its early development in Italy and only later did it spread beyond the Alps to France, central Europe, the Low Countries, and England. The central tenet of the humanists was the revival of classical learning, the rediscovery, so to speak, of Latin and Greek literature, of the classical models and classical values.

Humanism was an integral part of the larger movement that is commonly called the Renaissance. I like to think of this period, roughly 1300 to 1600, as the decline of an old culture and the emergence of a new. When I speak of a culture or way of life I mean two things: a set of values indicating what is deemed good, desirable, worth sacrificing for; and an Establishment or power élite, a hierarchy of leaders and followers, of those who tell others what to do and those who obey. You may, if you will, call this a pecking order.

The medieval period at its height represented a rich and varied culture, well adapted to the social, political, religious, and economic environment of the time, and organized around certain magnificent institutions, such as the Church, the Holy Roman Empire, the feudal system. The values in religion, politics, economics, art, science, social customs—and medicine— were coherent and held the allegiance of the mass of people. Pagan values had been for the most part rejected. The prevailing attitude was dogmatic and authoritarian, the intellectual activity largely rationalistic and analytic within a relatively closed circle. Medicine shared in this trend, which shaped both its theories and practice.

But the medieval culture which reached its pinnacle in the thirteenth century failed to keep pace with the changing conditions. Increase in knowledge made necessary new patterns of thinking. The old structure of ideas, of values, and of power was no longer adaptive. The changes that took place were extraordinarily complex, especially in the evaluation of what was good and desirable. There was an interaction or "feedback," so that new events produced new attitudes and standards, and these, in turn, brought about new events. The old standards no longer held allegiance; new adventures, new desires, new thoughts and values conflicted with the old; furthermore, there was a new struggle for power. We can think of a new culture emerging, by which I mean, again, the establishment of a new set of values and the setting up of new bases of power—a dethronement of the old pecking order and setting up a new one.

In this process the humanists represent a small and quite specific group. When we think of Renaissance humanists, we think of Petrarch and Boccaccio and Ariosto, Bruni and Valla, Erasmus and Thomas More. These, however, were only a few of the best known. A vast number of poets and philosophers and men of letters, historians, scholars, politicians, most of them relatively obscure, almost forgotten today, devoted themselves to classical learning and classical ideals. Humanism comprised not a profession or occupation, but rather an attitude and an interest. It is not surprising that many physicians of the era are numbered among the humanists.

The British physician Thomas Linacre will serve as an example. He lived from 1460 (or 1461) to 1524 and thus spanned the high period of humanist development. His early education in England took place in what was essentially a medieval atmosphere, for the new classical learning and the development of printing were much less advanced in England than on the Continent. In 1484 Linacre was admitted a fellow of All Souls College in Oxford, and in 1487 he went to Italy, probably to accompany an embassy from Henry VIII to the Pope. For some twelve years Linacre remained in Italy. He absorbed the classical tradition at its very source, got to know the great scholars of the time, and shared in their work. Linacre studied Greek with the best masters, paying particular attention to Aristotle and Galen, and he is said to be the first Englishman who studied these men in the original Greek. This was the period

when, with the development of printing, scholars were busy editing manuscripts for publication and making translations from the original Greek into Latin. Thus they could bring uncorrupted texts, either in Greek or in Latin, to the educated European.

While in Italy Linacre studied medicine at Padua and received his M.D. degree in 1496. When he returned to England, he became the first Englishman to have an international reputation in the new learning, and he was one of the small group of scholars who spread the new knowledge of Greek in Great Britain. In the practice of medicine he acquired a great reputation, for he was called to the court of Henry VII as court physician and also as tutor to the royal family. His various writings include translation of Greek medical and scientific works, particularly some of the Galenic texts, and also two books on Latin grammar. Linacre is best known today as the founder of the Royal College of Physicians, chartered by King Henry VIII in 1518.

I must emphasize that Linacre was not a radical reformer, but a conservative with some new ideas of proper standards. Fifteenth-century medicine was founded on the teachings of the ancients. Linacre wanted to recover these in all their purity and eliminate the corruption and uncertainty that had accrued in the Middle Ages. These defects, thought the humanists, were due to inadequate knowledge of the original sources. Medicine would immediately improve with recourse to the original sources.

A physician who went to Italy, studied Greek, and had first-hand acquaintance with the original classic texts, quickly acquired a great reputation when he returned home. We may draw a comparison to the colonial physicians in eighteenth-century America who went to Edinburgh to study medicine and then returned to the colonies; or, in the early twentieth century, to the American physicians who pursued postgraduate studies in Vienna and Berlin. The physicians who studied at the sources of medical progress immediately had a great advantage over those who did not.

As a second humanist physician I will mention Rabelais, the immortal creator of *Gargantua* and *Pantagruel*. He was a priest, a sound classical scholar, and also a physician who enjoyed considerable reputation. Virtually nothing is known of his early life, even the year of his birth. Most authorities accept 1490 as the date, although 1483 and 1495 have also been alleged. We know that he was a Franciscan monk, then became a Benedictine, and then abandoned his order to become a secular priest. He entered the medical school at Montpellier in 1531 and in a few months received the degree of bachelor of medicine. In 1532 he moved to Lyons and served as physician to the Hôtel Dieu, and lectured on anatomy. He edited works of Hippocrates and Galen, as well as other medical texts. At this time, in addition to his active medical work and studies in the classical medical texts, he was also working on his great literary masterpieces, *Pantagruel* and *Gargantua*.

He later returned to the Benedictine order, took the degree of doctor of medicine at Montpellier (1537). We know that he lectured on Hippocrates and conducted anatomical demonstrations with, we can assume, judging by his various medical activities, a considerable degree of competence. The details of his life are extremely complicated since the sources are confused, fragmentary, sometimes contradictory. For our purposes his various travels and conflicts are irrelevant, nor need we be concerned here with literary details.

Rabelais died in 1553, one of the great figures of Renaissance letters and an outstanding humanist, learned in classical Greek and Latin. According to the concepts of his time he, like the other medical humanists, advanced medicine by translating and editing classical texts. From our standpoint his great contribution to our cultural heritage lay in the field of letters, not medicine. In *Gargantua* and *Pantagruel* his satire exposes to us the defects of the educational, religious, and social environments. As a satirist he helped to bring about a new order, as a physician he did not. He was a medical conservative although, as we have seen, the attempt to expound the original old sources represented the progressive movement. The fact that he was a priest plays no part in our evaluation.

The third humanist physician I want to mention is the Englishman John Caius, who lived from 1510 to 1573. Born in Norwich, he was educated at Cambridge, then left England to study medicine at Padua where he got his degree in 1541. During his stay at Padua, Caius lived in the same house with Vesalius for a period of eight months. But despite this close contact, Caius, according to Clark,[3] never accepted Vesalius' innovations.

Nevertheless, Caius was an outstanding example of the new learning. He studied the original Greek medical texts, and like the other great humanists, translated works of Hippocrates and Galen into Latin. When he returned to England after further travels, he became one of the leading medical practitioners and was court physician to King Edward VI, Queen Mary, and Queen Elizabeth. As a fellow of the College of Physicians he took a prominent part in its affairs and was its president for many years. His was a strong hand and he used his powers to maintain medical orthodoxy. From his medical practice he amassed a large fortune and by his gifts to Cambridge University he raised Gonville Hall, where he had been a fellow, to the rank of College. This was named Gonville and Caius College, and he served as its master for almost twenty years.

Caius, however, did more than merely look to the past. Although a firm traditionalist, he had a strong interest in contemporary medicine and his most valuable writing (from our viewpoint) was his description of the so-called sweating sickness, epidemic at that time. This excursion into close personal study of a disease and its attendant phenomena represents a rather different facet, one that we might call a turning from the past to the present. And then, in addition to his work on a contemporary disease, Caius wrote a methodical study of British dogs, an indication of interest in nature, or what we might call natural history—rather a far cry from humanistic medicine.

I have touched briefly on three Renaissance physicians, covering a span of somewhat over one hundred years. These men, so different in many ways, had much in common, particularly their attempt to improve medicine by recovering and making available the classic texts of antiquity. This, of course, involved a deep knowledge of Greek and Latin and a profound scholarship. A further point of similarity was the breadth of their interests apart from their medical studies—Linacre with Latin grammars; Rabelais with his masterpieces of satire and humor, written in the vernacular; Caius with a text on British dogs. All these men were classical scholars but they were also quite aware of the present. They all left a deep imprint on the ongoing current of life —whether through the powerful College of Physicians or the study of a raging epidemic, or broad humor and brilliant satire.

The humanist physicians were Renaissance men, with many talents. Like the humanists in other fields they represented for the most part an aristocratic focus—intellectually and culturally privileged, devoted to gracious living. They rejected the medieval values. While for the most part they favored the classical values, they did not ignore the present. Yet in their concern with classical values they did neglect one major current that was soon to dominate Western culture—the current that we call science, better known then as "natural philosophy."

The humanists, like most thinking men of the fifteenth and sixteenth centuries, were highly dissatisfied with the contemporary way of life and its decayed ideals. In the rebellion against such corruption and the authority which lay behind it, the humanists sought their remedy in the distant past and in the culture of Greece and Rome. Others, however, equally dissatisfied, looked to nature. Such men were not aristocratic. This group represents not the armchair thinkers or scholars in their closets, but active doers with an empirical approach, who traveled and explored, who dissected and peered into nature's secrets, who worked with their hands, devising new methods and seeking new explanations. Some showed considerable concern for theory, others not; but they were one and all looking forward to the future rather than backward to the classical past.

For a comparison with our humanist physicians I would mention briefly two of the nonhumanists of the same period— Paracelsus, who lived from 1494 to 1541 and thus is quite comparable to Rabelais; and Ambroise Paré, who lived from 1510 to 1590, and thus is contemporary with Caius.

Paracelsus, or to give him his full name,

Philippus Aureolus Theophrastus Bombast of Hohenheim, called Paracelsus, was a rebel against authority. His attitude, I believe, was probably rooted in a deep-seated personality disorder, for he was quarrelsome and antagonistic, constantly traveling, never able to adapt to any one locale.

We have little knowledge about his early life and education. He knew some Latin but did not, apparently, have real facility in this language and he taught and wrote for the most part in the vernacular. He at least visited many famous universities but we do not know how long, if at all, he studied at them. We do not even know whether he had a medical degree. He did, however, serve for a while as an army surgeon, and throughout his life he traveled widely, practicing medicine, writing extensively, and acquiring considerable reputation.

Paracelsus set himself apart from the medical establishment. In 1527, while lecturing in Basle, he publicly burned the works of Galen and Avicenna, to indicate his rejection of traditional medicine. His own doctrines are extremely complex and cannot be expounded here. Suffice to indicate three key points. He had intense concern with concrete observation. The physician, he taught, must learn from the book of nature and not from the ancient authors whose books were not sufficiently founded on observation. Then, he was deeply involved in what we might call the spiritual aspects of nature. He perceived an essential unity of all natural entities and processes and was greatly concerned with the interrelationship of the microcosm and the macrocosm. Then, he emphasized the importance of chemistry in the understanding of the universe and of man. The vital processes of man, he taught, were essentially chemical. He introduced many chemical remedies into medical practice.

Despite the obscurities of his writings and their many contradictions, Paracelsus was a truly seminal figure in medical history who, even though he made many false turnings, markedly influenced the progress of medicine and helped to direct it into its present form. We can readily perceive the sharp contrast between Paracelsus the rebel and Linacre or Caius, the humanists.

An even sharper contrast, however, we see between Ambroise Paré and the humanists. Paré (1510-1590) had a meager education, never learned Latin, and had no pretentions to scholarship in the classical tradition. He was a barber-surgeon, belonging to a craft rather than a learned profession. His training, however, was excellent and the great military activity of the sixteenth century offered him vast scope for his abilities. His great contributions to surgery are well known and resulted from his native genius, independent mind, and inquiring spirit. He was concerned with the teachings of experience rather than with authority, and because he questioned and doubted, observed for himself and did not fear innovation, he was able to advance the art of surgery to new heights.

Paré wrote a great deal—in French, not Latin—and exerted a tremendous influence. Through independent observation, attention to natural phenomena, he showed the medical world the road to progress. He represented what we may call the nonintellectual tradition, the craftsman and technologist who manipulated nature and gained thereby an understanding of nature.

Humanism does indeed represent a revolt, resting on pervasive dissatisfaction and a striving toward something better. Dissatisfaction, of course, always exists, in what we may call "normal" amounts, but in some periods of history it builds up to a high intensity, over a broad base. Then it can bring about substantial change. This happened in the Renaissance.

By the fifteenth century the medieval culture, splendid indeed in its prime, was becoming decayed and sterile. New insights and a fresh approach were needed. In their search the discontented sought to break the limiting bonds and find new ways to achieve the better life, and this striving took many forms, went off in many directions. The humanists, particularly the medical humanists, tried to bring about an improvement through an escape to the past.

The humanist physicians felt that they had found a new method, and in a sense they did, for paradoxical as it may seem, the past is ever new. Whoever regards the past always sees it through eyes different from his neighbor's, or from his predecessor's. The past, while showing this paradoxical novelty, nevertheless has stability, so that a return to the past is in essence the conservative approach.

Once the ancient texts were recovered to a reasonable degree and the conservative ideals partly reestablished, then what? Were the humanists to stand still? Or if not, where were they to go? The scholasticism which the humanists rejected had failed to adapt to new demands and had decayed into logical quibbling and verbal trifling. The humanists, substituting a new set of ideals, met a comparable fate. The humanist devotion to the classics and the scorn for the medieval tradition were highly beneficial for a while, but soon came to a dead end. Virtually all historians comment on the bad side effects of the Renaissance humanism and the degeneration it soon underwent. Devotion to Ciceronian Latin could not restore vitality to what was really archaic. Vulgar Latin and vernacular languages were far more vital forms of expression, but were looked down upon. Classi-

cal Latin became more polished and refined but had less and less to say. The later humanists fell victim to pedantry; concern with form took precedence over substance and led to sterilty. The humanists who condemned scholastic authority and domination of the church, themselves bowed before an equal tyranny—the authority of the ancients. Such is the fate of the conservatism which, for whatever reason, fails to make substantive progress.

In the Renaissance, as we have seen, an alternative escape from scholasticism lay along the road of natural philosophy, which looked forward rather than backward. By the seventeenth century science was making enormous strides, and by that time the humanist movement had pretty much disintegrated. But it had accomplished a great deal. First of all, the humanists had evolved a critical sense. This critical acumen may have been verbal, concerned with documents rather than biological or physical phenomena, but it represented an attitude that pervaded the entire area.

Then, the humanists inculcated a love for the classical ideals and forms. The classical tradition dominated the sixteenth and seventeenth centuries, even though it turned into the baroque and the rococo. As examples, Corneille, Racine, and the Louvre, illustrate the working out of the classical trends, as do the defenders of the ancients, in the so-called "Battle of the Ancients and the Moderns." Obviously, we cannot credit humanism as such with the whole unrolling of post-Renaissance classical development, but the humanists did provide a great deal of the motive power.

The humanists provided a foundation for the advances of others but their own tenets, in the narrower sense, did not share in this advance. The humanists rebelled against the sterile forms that resulted from the decay in medieval culture. They sought new insight and a fresh approach—which they found, to some extent. But these in turn became sterile and decayed.

During this period science was making continuous progress. Even in the fifteenth and sixteenth centuries we can see the conflict between the study of nature on the one hand and humanistic learning on the other. To the sixteenth century we may not want to apply the term "the two cultures," but the germs of the separation were certainly present and growing.

I need not stress the enormous advances science has made in the past four centuries nor the transformations it has wrought. Science has, perhaps, been too successful, has assumed such a dominating position that its very dominance may entail its own destruction. Even to the casual observer there is visible crumbling around the edges. Whether the foundations are still sound we cannot at present tell. But I personally believe we today are in a position comparable to the late Middle Ages, with science taking the place of the church, the scientist of the priest. I believe that our institutions, as with those in the fifteenth century, are no longer sufficiently adaptive to changing circumstances. As in the fifteenth century there is a deeply felt need for change, and this need, among the hardy, is being translated into disruptive action—into radical activity.

But today's conservatives want to recover the values of the past, the values which pertain to man as something distinct from nature. Today it is quite difficult to separate man and his activities from the rest of nature, but the separation still has validity. Humanists today continue to emphasize the qualitative values of life, the specific and the particular, whereas the scientists strive after universals and quantifications.

We find humanistic values all around us, in our literature and art and history, in personal communications and empathy, in ethical standards and the sense of human dignity, in the esthetic appreciation and striving for excellence. These are the eternal ingredients of humanism. Classical humanism came to the fore, in the Renaissance, as a reaction against a decaying dominant culture. Humanism is again coming to the fore today as our own dominant culture is weakening. Let us use the humanistic stirrings of mankind to build a new Renaissance.

REFERENCES

1. Stalcup, S.A.: Relevance today and tomorrow in medical education—a forum with a purpose. *Calif Med, 112*:6, 1970.
2. Stead, E. A.: Medical education and practice. *Ann Intern Med, 72*:271-274, 1970.
3. Clark, Sir G.: *A History of the Royal College of Physicians.* London, Oxford University Press, vol. 1, p. 107, 1964.

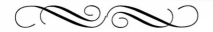

Essay II

Man's Inhumanity to His Great Men*

HEBBEL E. HOFF, M.D., Ph.D.

DR. HICKEY, DR. MCGOVERN, DR. BURNS, DR. TRUMAN; distinguished sons of Osler, and his descendents reaching into the third and fourth generations. As it now devolves on me to be the first to speak at this Symposium on Humanism in Medicine, let me say that at no time in recent history has the subject ever been less of a sentimental reunion of like-minded people to reminisce on the pleasant things of the past, or more of an occasion to approach man's real being, assess his position in the whole of nature, and prepare ourselves for the plunge we must take in the void of the future. In that plunge man looks more like he does in the only figure I will show you, traced on the walls of one of the French caves some sixteen thousand years ago, where there was little talk of man's conquest of nature, and the fearful horns and the hot eyes of Death often stared down at a fragile man, his spears ineffective and broken and his newest invention, a spear thrower, fallen

from his grasp. You will note too something quite human about this man; he saw himself even then as quite different from the rest of nature. The Bull is realistic and breathes a fierce dynamism—Picasso has never done better—but man depicts himself as a thing of straw and matchsticks; he is an enigma to himself, but he shows his defiance in the face of death with his erect phallus.

Yesterday morning I stayed away from the office to see the first of the "Today" programs on the ruin that man has made of his environment. It was a pretty complete indictment of man's behavior. Man was told that he had an utterly false concept of his position at the apex of the living world, at the highest mark of evolution, and as the creature for whom the world was made. He was accused of alienating himself from nature and losing sight of his place in the natural world. He was directed to recast his philosophies and redirect the full force of the new technologies of which he is now a master to protect and not exploit his environment, and to preserve in a planned ecological balance the whole of nature and the world around him. It was thorough indictment indeed, and it was a monumental challenge.

You will perceive easily enough the paradox involved in this proposal, because to accomplish this, man will have to take an even more important position in nature and

*Supported in part by USPH-LM00453-04 from the National Library of Medicine

11

instead of living as they say *on* nature, he will have to remake the world in his image and treat the whole of it as a natural environment to be husbanded. In the philosophy and the technology of all this there is no one else to accomplish it but man; man then will have to assume an even more important role in nature. Is the parable of the good shepherd weakened because as every one knows the sheep is fleeced or eaten?

The greatest task that man has to face in the future is thus to decide who he is and what his relationship with the world is going to be. Whatever way this turns out, we can be sure to see an even greater involvement of man in nature and a greater degree of control over nature. This can no longer follow along the discredited line of the conquest of nature, about which we have heard only too much, but toward the discovery of the nature of man and his reunion with nature.

Man has indeed passed through two stages of this relation, the first one the fear of nature; it is implicit in the illustration and in many forms it still survives. From his fear grew the drive to conquer what he feared most. Are we ready to forget our fears and so forget our need to conquer? Probably not completely, and probably not quite yet. When the time comes, however, it must be man who does it, for man in one respect is different from the rest of nature; he alone has the power of cultural evolution so that he can, however slowly, change his cultural inheritance and adapt his behavior to meet the problems that face him.

My own approach today concerns a minor aspect of the whole; it deals with the tendency man has to turn his great men into gods and then to turn around and expect them to behave like God. This is, no doubt, part of his cultural heritage from Mesopotamia where the idea of the great polar opposites seems first to have developed, of light and dark, of cold and hot, of wet and dry, of man and god, of good and bad, that so permeate our thinking that we can hardly think of one thing except in terms of its opposite.

I mentioned its ancient origin simply so that we may ask ourselves how quickly can we change imbedded cultural patterns and displace the patterns of thinking and behaving that now beset us. It will not be easy. If we cannot indeed escape changing our great men into gods as happened to Imhotep and Aesculapius or canonizing them as the Middle Ages did with Galen and the Russians tried to do with Pavlov, perhaps we could revise our estimate of how gods should behave; Amphitryon and Gideon come to mind as possible models.

It is said that a group of friends once called on Heraclitus, who, as you know carried over into Grecian philosophy something of this idea of opposites, and found him busy in the kitchen. (There is some difficulty about the translation of the word kitchen and some people read it dung heap. This would make it better from the standpoint of this account and maybe this is how the dung heap got into Heraclitus' history.) The visitors were embarrassed and hesitated to enter, but Heraclitus called out saying, "Don't be embarrassed, come in, there are gods even here." What he meant, of course, is that no matter how we approach a phenomenon of nature and however small and insignificant this small area may be, to illuminate it will cast light into farther perspectives and some progress can be made. It is not unnatural that such a man would look upon *change* as the truth to be found.

As an example of our tendency to demand greater than human qualities in our great men, let me mention the remarkable collection of essays about Sir William on the fiftieth anniversary of his death. In it was a delicate apology about Osler's lack of genuine eminence as a scientist. I suppose we would have to admit that he was not, but I was stirred to react strongly to it in the words of Heraclitus; there were gods in the laboratory of pathology, there were gods in the wards of the hospital, there were gods in Osler's consulting room. Not all the gods of medicine frequent full time medicine and the Flexner Report. Why then demand that a man seek other gods someplace else? So were we to lay down rules of human achievement the first would be that a man should be evaluated for what he is and for what he accomplishes, and not for what he is not and does not do.

Let me now introduce, with somewhat less confidence that you will accept them, two further ideas that go something like this. A great man can indeed have great defects, and he can be great despite those defects. This I believe most of you will accept. Now let me propose a third thought, which is, that perhaps some of those very qualities of character and personality that seem to be his greatest defects and have handicapped a man in many, many ways, are at the same time the very wellsprings of his greatness, and that if we took away these qualities then the dynamic core of the *man* would disintegrate. Some of these we readily excuse as unusual foibles or eccentricities; we can think of E. Y. Davis, in Osler's life, for instance, even though we feel instinctively that there is much more to E. Y. Davis than that. This we have learned to accept in art. We have not learned to accept it in medicine, though I think we must come to it.

Let me review a few examples that many would not accept as evidence. First let us consider our old and dear friend Theophrastus Bombast von Hohenheim, otherwise known as Paracelsus. He was certainly guilty of the free and frequent use of four letter words or their German equivalent whenever he wanted people to understand clearly what he meant. He was equally guilty of coining the most abstruse, bastard Greek-Latin words when he did not want to let people know quite what he meant. He was, in our modern terminology, a graduate school bum, moving from one university to another. He argued with his professors, he never took examinations; he certainly practiced without a license; he overcharged and quarreled with his patients: he frequented taverns; he had no respect at all for Galen and Hippocrates; he was a mystic, an antibaptist, a cabalist and an astrologer, among other things, while remaining true to the Catholic faith, and he antagonized the good members of the establishment in city after city. Such were the Fuggers who had a monopoly on the importation of guaiac which they sold to relieve the symptoms of the French disease. Paracelsus touched their pocketbooks to the quick by preaching that their product was utterly useless for the purpose. It was not, but that is incidental. From this unlikely source came the beginnings of chemistry in medicine, the concept of the natural healing of wounds, the first account of occupational disease, and the idea of local biochemical disease producing local anatomical change.

Let us next mention Johannes Baptista Van Helmont, quoting the following evaluation written when he died: "This man was a wicked Flemish rascal who died insane a few months ago. He did nothing of value. I have seen all that he has done. This man had in mind only a medicine full of chemical and empirical secrets and to overthrow it more quickly he came out strongly against blood letting, for the lack of which he died mad."

So wrote Guy Patin to his friend Spohn in Lyon. In the same letter, to show the conventional position, Guy Patin told of two cures he had effected only recently. One was a man whom he had bled sixty four times in eight months and the second a seven year old boy whom he had bled thirteen times in fifteen days. There can be no doubt that Van Helmont failed to follow the best examples in medical practice in his community! This unorthodoxy was documented in his earliest paper on the magnetic cure of wounds, which managed to get him in trouble both with the faculty and with the church. At the same time, he was careless and even contemptuous of good literary scholarship, writing that in the multitude of books there is nowhere comfort of knowledge, but vain promises, abuses, and very many errors.

He had indeed learned too well Heraclitus' words that the almighty gods are everywhere and Aristotle's modification of it to emphasize the comparative study of nature when he wrote and admonished people "in a like manner we ought not to be abashed but boldly to enter upon our researches concerning animals of every sort, knowing that in not one of them is nature or beauty lacking." He was following the admonition of the great Rhenish philosopher and preacher Tauler who wrote, "The great masters of Paris read big books and turn the pages. This is good, but others read the living book where everything lives eternally and turn to the heavens and earth to read the wonderful works of God." Clearly, he must have read Nicholas of Cusa who remonstrated with the Orator in his little book *The Idiot,* remarking about this matter of books and the opinions of authority (this from a prince of the church in 1450!):

The opinion of authority hath perverted thee and made thee like an horse which being free by nature is by art tied to the manger with a halter where he eats nothing but what is given him, for thy understanding being bound to the authority of books is fed with strange and not natural foods. This is what I said, that thou art led by authority and so deceived. Somebody hath written this and thou believest him, but I say unto you that wisdom cryeth out from the streets.

We can trace this line then from Heraclitus to Tauler and many others and on to Osler when he tells us about the books which were so dear and close to him that he said they were the compass of his life. But we must always remember that he added, that to live with books alone is like never putting out to sea. Perhaps much of what we have to do in the future is to get on with the job in the kitchen and be confident that gods are exactly there.

Then there was Luigi Galvani, an old friend of mine, surely one of the least scholarly of all professors. He apparently read the literature, but very little, and not deeply; he followed no clearly defined scientific method, he did not know how to design an experiment and much of his life was devoted to attempting to prove a truth that he had conceived of *a priori*. The point, of course, is that this is just what he did.

The three crucial experiments he performed were universal failures in some respects. The first experiment was a laboratory reproduction of Mahon's phenomenon of the "returning stroke" that had been thoroughly worked over some years before Galvani noted it.

The second experiment, from which he concluded on the existence of an animal electricity from the contraction of a muscle when it and its nerve were touched by the two extremities of an arc formed from two dissimilar metals, was quickly proven wrong. Absolutely irrefutable logic shows that if the arc is simply supposed to be a metallic connection between the inside and outside of his hypothetical Leyden jar in the muscle, why are two metals required? Any single metal should do. It was, of course, washed clear out of consideration by Volta's multiplication of added layers of dissimilar metals to produce the battery, whose sparks convinced the most skeptical that the instrument actually produced electricity.

But in this third experiment, stimulating a nerve by the current that exists between an injured and a non-injured area of the muscle, he did indeed come to a demonstration in which contraction was produced without metal and from the muscle itself. The discovery came too late to afford Galvani any great personal satisfaction, but in due course of time it was proven that this was the result of a natural electrical phenomenon; here was the beginning of animal electricity.

It has not been given to many men to found two new sciences, yet the science of current electricity and the science of bioelectric phenomena had their beginnings with this man who did all of the wrong things except live in his laboratory and follow the lead of the experiments which nature provided him.

I need not say much about John Hunter, except to tell a story that relates to him. Some years ago when John Fulton died, I was asked to write an appreciation of his contributions to physiology. To give some idea of his versatility and of the many things to which his genius led him, I began to write down his manifold interests one after another as they had crowded upon him. First on one sheet, then on to another, and another, the topics which he had dealt with in his career flowed upon the paper. Cere-bral localization, reflex activities, the function of the muscle spindle, cortical control of the autonomic nervous system, the function of the prefrontal lobes; we could go on and on like this. Then as I kept adding to this catalogue and began to get the feeling of the breadth and depth of this great person, I realized that I was unconsciously imitating a biographer who had done the same thing for Hunter, and that I was merely copying his technique.

So I came to understand that in many, many ways, John Fulton and John Hunter shared something in their vigorous exploration of nature without too much worry about its proper category, whether it was physiological, anatomical or pathological; versatile minds could encompass it all. So I wrote it down and sent a copy of the rough draft to another Fulton friend. By return mail I got back a frantic letter: "For heaven's sakes remove the reference associating John Fulton and Hunter; Fulton was a gentleman."

He was indeed, and I suppose you could really say Hunter was not. He was not a very good scientist in some respects, and responsible for some very poor human experimentation with himself as the subject, which made things very difficult for him years later. But somehow or another Hunter finds himself a nodal point through which the whole of surgery passes. Somehow or another the crude elements of the experiments on man that he was the first to attempt appeared in an almost perfect form in the experiments of his pupil Jenner. Let us not then worry too much about whether Hunter was a gentleman.

I do not need to be too concerned about any of these people, because the world has, by and large, done them justice, or approximately so. If he needed defense Paracelsus would have pulled out his long sword and flailed about him shouting loud German oaths while being sure to belabor his people only with the flat. Helmont acquiesced to the judgment of his church and university and stayed in virtual house arrest working busily and continuing his career. Hunter could storm into his wife's drawing room and throw everybody out because they were bothering his studies, and not worry about them, or his wife, too much. Galvani had his wife Lucia and that was apparently worth the rest of the world to him. Then, too, all of them had that total absorption in their work and needed to pay but little attention to what the world was thinking.

Finally, I believe they had something that is the greatest of all gifts to man; throughout the whole of their lives they could keep working, constantly occupied with new ideas and new projects. Even when Hunter began to see the world as tilted downhill or when he saw things in miniature or in grossly inflated form because of his cerebral disarray, and although he knew that whenever he became angry he threatened his own life, he nevertheless continued to be vigorous, thinking and productive.

Let me conclude, then, by introducing a problem that has never been solved, bringing it to you only as outline for further work. It concerns what is perhaps the greatest American contribution to medicine, in which nevertheless the individuals involved were totally ruined by their discovery and could thereafter never pull their lives together in an effective continuing career. This is the story of the three remarkable people who discovered ether anesthesia; to this day no one has carefully picked his way through the whole of it.

The basic outlines of the story, you all know. Simply and quickly told, on December 10, 1844, a young traveling lecturer came to Hartford to stage an exhibit of nitrous oxide inhalation. This youth, Gardner Quincy Colton must have been a very remarkable fellow, the only one of the whole group who saw himself in true light, calling himself only a messenger of the gods; certainly he was all of that. He too was the only man who profited by the invention of anesthesia, somewhat later opening painless dentistry establishments over the country and making a fair share of money by giving nitrous oxide as a dental anesthetic. He invested most of it in Florida real estate during the first Florida boom and died broke and happy; all the turmoil passed over him.

He had been a medical student in New York City, and as medical students did, he had learned of nitrous oxide and experimented with its exhilarating effects. Making up an ample supply, he gave a public lecture and demonstration of its effects, earning some five hundred dollars thereby. A good Yankee, the very next day he changed from medical student to professor and started to spread his message throughout New England.

New England at that time was still encrusted with its puritanical ideas, yet trying to break out of its confines, and had invented the compromise of the visiting educational lecturer who, on the basis of a scientific or other informative lecture, would present something interesting and entertaining. Colton's lecture and demonstration must have been both in full measure. In much the same way in those days (and ours too), the parson or the preacher could speak of hell and damnation and give semi-explicit statements about the type of sin available in the larger social centers which would entertain, frighten and shock the congregation, but yet was perfectly unexceptionable because it was done in church and for the best of interests. So people came to such educational lectures in considerable numbers; it was their substitute for the theatre.

At the session that night, or perhaps the next morning, there came a twenty seven year old dentist, Horace Wells, a gentle soul and one of the nicest people imaginable, married to a delightful girl, Elizabeth Wales. He had had and was to have many ups and downs in his life. An amateur inventor, he hoped to make his fortune but like many others never quite accomplished it.

At that meeting, a young apothecary's apprentice, Samuel Cooley, took the gas, became excited, ran around the stage, barked and bloodied his shins and showed no feeling of pain. Immediately, in a flash of insight, Wells saw in nitrous oxide the answer to painless surgery. He recruited Colton, went to his colleague Riggs, had some more gas prepared and inhaled it while Riggs painlessly extracted a wisdom tooth. The next week Wells assembled the necessary apparatus, learned how to make the gas, began to give it to his patients and in a few weeks was practicing anesthesia in dentistry. Word leaked out to the press in Boston, where a single reference stated that news from the West spoke of an interesting medical discovery.

To introduce the idea properly, Wells soon carried his discovery to Boston. Here was a friend, a former partner and a former pupil, William Morton. He was a dentist who had learned his dentistry from Wells or somewhere else; it is not even known if he ever studied it formally anywhere, but he was practicing it. He had gone to Boston to open a dentist's office and to enter Harvard Medical School as a student as part of the bargain he had made with his wife's father, who not considering the practice of dentistry quite good enough for his daughter's husband, had approved of the marriage on the condition that he would enroll in Harvard Medical School with a view to upgrading his profession. So he had, and at his friend Well's request he arranged with John Collins Warren, his professor of surgery, for Wells to give a demonstration before the class. As you know, it failed miserably. Students laughed, jeered and cried humbug!, driving Wells off the platform, out of Boston and out of dentistry, into such a complete depression that he may never have recovered completely.

The idea of anesthesia, however unsuccessfully presented by Wells, clearly must have stuck in Morton's mind, for on the night of September 30, 1846, Morton dropped in to visit his old professor, Charles T. Jackson. Not a very old professor, he was only forty-one, but he seems to be a particularly knowledgeable kind of professor who knew many answers in many fields and was always willing to give advice. Morton had boarded in Jackson's house the year before and his first son had been born there, so there was close attachment between them.

Morton carried with him a gas bag, saying he had an apprehensive patient coming that evening and wondered if by filling the bag with room air for her to breathe, she might be mesmerized and permit the proposed extraction. Jackson, puttering around the laboratory, advised him, almost as an aside, not to bother with such an attempt but to try sulfuric ether. According to the best evidence this is all he said, and that is exactly what Morton did. He stopped by the druggist, bought a bottle, and continued on to his office, where he found a patient waiting, one Ebenezer Frost, not at all the person he was expecting. He poured ether liberally on his handkerchief, put his patient to sleep, extracted the tooth, and after he awoke induced him to sign a testimonial about the painless procedure. He brought it down to the newspaper office that very night, and the next morning there was an advertisement for painless dentistry. After no more than two hectic weeks of dental anesthesia there was the surgery at the Massachusetts General Hospital and the world had anesthesia.

This brought new problems. Morton truly thought he should make some money from the discovery. He designed inhalers; he added oil of lavender to disguise the odor of ether and proposed to sell it as a material called Letheon; he proposed to license surgeons to give it, and to sell inhalers; for a while it looked like it was going to be a very good thing. Jackson, hearing of this, recognized his own contribution, went to his lawyer and suggested he should have a part in it. Morton was agreeable and the two jointly applied for and were awarded a patent.

In Hartford, Wells, seeing the newspaper accounts, recognized what appeared to be his own discovery. Jackson and Morton quarreled about the division of the European royalties, none of which ever materialized. Soon these three people, closely associated as friends could ever be, were now totally alienated, speaking of each other as that impostor and ignoramus Morton, or this rascal Wells, or this greedy and unscrupulous Jackson. Naturally some bright surgeon very quickly smelled ether in Letheon. Morton in fact had revealed to John Collins Warren exactly what the material was—there had been no attempt to deceive Collins—and one way or another everybody quickly knew that the active element was sulfuric ether and that it could be bought anywhere. It was as quickly found that when dropped on a towel it operated just as well as with a complicated

patent inhaler. So Morton found it virtually impossible to sell licenses; he sold few if any inhalers, and he was unable to sell any Letheon. Nobody derived any money out of it whatever, but all received an ample budget of ill will trying to get it.

It then developed that Congress had established a practice of making grants to those who had made notable contributions to society through useful inventions, and each of the three protagonists, independently and on his own account attempted to induce Congress to reward what each considered to be his own independent discovery. Each time a bill would come up to make an award to Morton, Wells' or Jackson's congressman would block it. The same fate awaited similar attempts by Wells or Jackson. In the end, nobody received anything from the Congress.

Wells was the first to suffer, as might be imagined, because his was the more sensitive nature. Moving to New York alone to establish himself as a professional anesthetist (and it is not known to what extent he did succeed in this role), he found himself alone in his room and lonely on the evening of January 21, 1848, the eve of his thirty-third birthday. Wells had acquired the habit of inhaling chloroform, one that other medical students and anesthesiologists also have acquired as with nitrous oxide and ether. That night after a few spells with chloroform, he and a friend went out carrying dropper bottles of sulphuric acid, with which it had become their custom as of other young men in town, to drop acid on the clothes of the prostitutes parading on Broadway. I need not go into the not very subterranean problems involved in why one would think of doing this, much less do it, but do it they did. The girls had identified them on previous occasions and were on the watch for them that night. As Wells dropped the acid the girls seized him and called for the police. That night he found himself in the Tombs on the eve of his thirty-third birthday, plunged again into an abyss of guilt and fear for the disgrace to his family and for his own sanity. So in the early hours of the next morning, fortifying himself with chloroform, he severed his left femoral artery, with the razor an accommodating warder had brought from his lodgings, and bled to death in his bed.

Morton and Jackson kept up an active vendetta, both receiving a good deal of credit and acclaim, though always clouded by the shadow of the other's claim.

Morton soon gave up Harvard Medical School, and before too long gave up dentistry, living a somewhat unsettled life trying to get help from one place or another, losing virtually everything in the process. On the night of July 12, 1868, he heard that Jackson had issued a new counterblast. Jackson was not without resources and had hired detectives who worked out in detail much of the chicanery that Morton had practiced while a young man in the West. This is a whole story in itself, but it suffices to say that one of the persons involved, and perhaps victimized, had stated in the public press that Morton was capable of any crime that did not demand physical courage. This being all uncovered by Jackson, Morton, worried about what was going to happen next, rushed to New York to meet with his lawyers and counter this newest attack.

Driving in Central Park with his wife to avoid the heat of the evening, he stopped the carriage near the small lake that is still there and walked over to it to cool himself. Here he had what must have been a cerebral accident, and died at the edge of the pond. A crowd collected, an ambulance was called and, as might still happen today in Central Park, while he was lying there somebody rifled his pockets of their modest contents. The ambulance brought him to St. Luke's Hospital where the surgeon identified the body, and calling the clerks and the students around it, remarked that they saw before them the man who had done more for humanity and more for helping human pain than any other man who had ever lived. His wife pulled from her purse the last remnants of his possessions, three medals he had been awarded in better times, and laying them on her husband's body remarked bitterly that these were all he ever received for it.

Morton's death was a great disappointment to Jackson. His great adversary was gone and public sympathy for him began to rise. His own family and friends must have worried about Jackson because he was prone, they thought, to claim discoveries of others for himself; perhaps also they saw in his contentiousness the beginnings of his subsequent mental breakdown. This may be why of all these three, history has dealt least well with Jackson. Back in 1832 he had been returning from Europe on a brig, the *Sully,* and in the long hours over the captain's table there had been the usual talk of all kinds of subjects. With his knowledge of chemistry and geology and electricity and much else he must have expounded freely on modern science.

One of the young people at the table remarked that since the new electrical fluid traveled so very rapidly, could one not arrange to send messages by its means? Jackson replied in the vein that it would be no trouble at all to send such messages. An electromagnet might be activated by a battery by means of a key at the end of a long stretch of wire, the circuit being completed through the ground. Pressing the key could activate the magnet to write out messages;

it might be possible to devise codes, etc. The young man suggested that on their return to New York they meet and construct a working model. Jackson was soon off on other subjects, being one of those persons perhaps to whom the idea is as good as reality, and he did not accept the suggestion, so the young man worked it out alone. His name was Samuel Morse, of course.

After the telegraph became a practical reality Jackson was often heard to claim that he had invented the telegraph. Now Jackson was also saying he had invented anesthesia; no one seemed to believe the whole of it. From contesting with Morton alive Jackson went on to reviling him when dead, and in time it became clear that he was deranged. Taken to the McLane Asylum, he spent there the last years of his life.

Here was a man who with two short declarations, "try electromagnetism" and "try ether," had given the original impetus to two of the greatest inventions in America of the nineteenth century, or perhaps of any time. Few would believe it. Here was a young dentist who had foreseen precisely the whole idea of anesthesia. It was taken from him because he failed in a critical demonstration. Here was Morton who was the dynamic and central force connecting Wells and Jackson, and who converted a vague suggestion into universal reality. Few

believed that he could have contributed anything essential because he was an ignorant dentist, and ignorant dentists simply do not make inventions. Furthermore, he had certainly had a checkered career as a gentle swindler throughout the West and this must have prevented him from doing anything worthwhile.

Neither in the advanced culture of Boston, or anywhere else, for that matter, was there anyone to see what today looks like an unbreakable chain linking these three people, welding their individual contributions into the whole that constitutes the discovery. Each had defects, but I believe we can see that their very defects, the sensitivity of Wells, the eagerness to exploit of Morton, and the dogmatic or pedantic way Jackson had of throwing off a suggestion, were the keys to the discovery. What were the most unpleasant and the most trialsome things about these people were in essence the things that gave discovery its life. I have tried to get this record straight, not with the expectation of finally assigning the credit the past demands, but because, if we are to create an environment of progress and invention in the future, we must turn to the true nature of man, so that we can understand the wellsprings of productivity and fertility and try to create and continue that kind of environment.

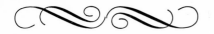

Osler & Halsted, a Contrast in Personalities

EMILE HOLMAN, M.D.

PROLOGUE

Patient care is undergoing a rapid change —whether for better or for worse is not at present foreseeable. The patient of today is in danger of being alienated by the technical straitjacket into which his doctors have thrust him.

The doctor in turn is in danger of being viewed as a sophisticated technician, concerned primarily with mindless but efficient machines, with electric and electronic devices, with chemical tests in wholesale lots, with gadgets innumerable, and with an impersonal catechism that obscures the all-important details of the patient's illness which it is supposed to enlighten. In this process, the doctor is losing his role as a sympathetic healer.

As the present trend continues, patient care inevitably becomes more depersonalized and dehumanized. In the meanwhile, humanism is becoming recognized as an indispensable and integral aspect of a patient's care. Osler so enriched the lives of his patients and of society in general with his deeply humanistic approach to society's ills, that he was recognized early as a prototype of what a physician should be.

We may well ask, what is humanism?

It connotes compassion, benevolence and charity. It implies human understanding, a social conscience, and a sympathetic attitude toward those in distress.

We are here today to explore the meaning of humanism, and to seek ways of re-infusing patient care with kindness, compassion, and sympathy.

Sir William Osler is universally credited with having been the leading physician and medical teacher of his day. Today he is presented also as the leading medical humanist of his time. Certain it is that, no matter where he lived—in Canada, in America, or in Britain; no matter where he taught, practiced, or wrote—his sterling qualities of character shone in highest brilliance. "Osler was a well nigh perfect example of the union of science and the humanities,"[5] wrote Sir Frederic Kenyon, one of Britain's great classical scholars.

In an introduction to Osler's address on "The Old Humanities and the New Science," Harvey Cushing wrote: "Sir William Osler was a man first—a physician and scholar afterward; and beneath his high spirits, his love of fun, lay an infinite compassion and tenderness toward his human kind."[5]

How and whence came this ardent humanist, this universally revered scientist? A brief review of the salient features of his life provides important clues.[2]

He was born in 1849 at Bond Head at the then edge of Ontario's wilderness, twenty-five miles from Toronto, the youngest boy of nine children of an Anglican missionary who served numerous parishes in twenty townships, travelling always on horseback. The mother of these nine children, born under the primitive conditions of the frontier, lived not only to celebrate her one hundredth birthday, but also to see three of her sons attain international fame, one as a lawyer, one as a banker, and one as a physician. Here one detects Osler's key possession: superior genes!

Young Willie early came under the salutary guidance of a Reverend Johnson who introduced him to the wonderful world to be seen under a microscope, and before the age of twenty this lad had written three papers on the diatomaceae, the infusoria, and the polyzoa found in Canadian waters. Although originally directed toward the clergy, he graduated from McGill Medical School in 1872, and spent the next two years in Europe studying under Virchow, Rokitansky, Jenner, and Burdon Sanderson. On his return at the ripe age of twenty-five, he was made professor of medical institutes at McGill which involved the teaching of physiology, pathology and histology. The students dubbed him the "Baby Professor."

A year later he was made pathologist to the Montreal General Hospital and in the next nine years he performed over nine hundred autopsies, the protocols of which filled five volumes, written in his own hand, carefully correlating the clinical picture with his own observations at the autopsy table. On the title page of one of these volumes he wrote: "Pathology is the basis for all true instruction in clinical medicine." These exacting and instructive experiences in the post-mortem room, many times repeated, undoubtedly provided the basis for the uncanny clinical sense which he displayed in later years.

In 1884 at the age of thirty-five he was made professor of medicine at the University of Pennsylvania, then considered the highest post in medicine in this hemisphere.

In the meantime Johns Hopkins of Baltimore, a Quaker who was not unwilling to make a dollar in the selling and bartering of liquor, had left his seven million dollar fortune for the founding of a university and a hospital.[7] Seven million dollars at that time bought what 130 million dollars would buy today. A bachelor, he sought advice how best to perpetuate his name. He was advised by a friend to found a university—there would always be students; by another friend to found a hospital—there would always be sick people; and so he founded both, each with its own endowment and its own board of trustees.

The construction of the hospital was begun in 1877, but was not completed until twelve years later, only the income of the endowment being used. This unique tactic was stipulated in Mr. Hopkins' will. The medical school itself did not open until 1893, four years later, and then only through the fortuitous interest of a group of prominent Baltimore women who offered the $500,000 necessary to finish the school on one condition: *that women be admitted on the same basis as men.* Dr. Welch, the dean, shied at the word "same" and wanted to change it to "equal," but the ladies would have none of it. The offer was accepted.

A second distinctive feature was the requirement of a bachelor of arts degree for admission to the medical school. Harvard followed suit eight years later. Such high standards of admission to the new school were set that Osler once remarked to Welch, the dean: "It's good you and I entered this school as professors—we never would have made it as students!"

A third unusual, and, at that time unique feature, was extension of the medical curriculum to four years beyond the degree of bachelor of arts.

The dominant influence in the new school besides Welch was Osler. These two impresarios were a great team, working harmoniously and effectively together with much amusing repartee between them. Osler's great respect for Welch is revealed in his comment that "Welch has a three-story intellect with an attic on top."

Osler laid the greatest emphasis first on the patient and second on the student. He abolished didactic lectures and made the student an integral part of the hospital organization. Said he modestly: "I hope my gravestone will bear only the statement: 'He brought medical students into the wards for bedside teaching'." In addition, he made the students responsible for the history of the patient's illness, for a complete physical examination, and for the simpler laboratory examinations. To us now, all this seems quite commonplace, but at that time it took vision, courage and faith to assign such important tasks to "mere" students. Osler himself was beset by the haunting fear that these innovations would be fought by the public and spurned by the medical profession. To his genuine relief, their acceptance by both was immediate and general, and they survive today as important keystones in medical education.

Osler was known as a therapeutic nihilist. He had no sympathy with random polypharmacy and relied a great deal on Mother Rest and Father Time. He was fond of quoting Oliver Wendell Holmes that if the entire pharmacopoeia were dumped into the ocean it would be good for the patients but very bad for the fishes!

He was an inspiring teacher of students for he himself remained a student to the very end. As MacCallum once wrote, ". . . he made frequent visits to the autopsy room, studying in death the puzzles he had helped solve, or failed to explain, during life." His influence on Johns Hopkins was incalculable. He set a pattern that is still an intimate part of the Hopkins of today.

It was at Oxford that I knew him, a gracious and generous host—especially to American doctors and students, a fascinating teacher, a profound student of the classics (he became president of the British Classical Association), and an enthusiastic medical historian and bibliophile, who in his lifetime collected 7,600 volumes, including 104 incunabula.

These manifold interests made his teaching a delight, replete with literary and historical allusions, and apt quotations. To him a patient was not a drunkard, he was a "disciple of Bacchus"; he was not a laborer but a "follower of Vulcan." If a victim of syphillis or gonorrhea, he was referred to in bedside conversation as "a devotee of Eros or Venus."

On ward rounds his diagnostic acumen was a constant cause for surprise and admiration. One Sunday morning, as he entered the ward his eye had rested only momentarily on the first patient when he exclaimed: "Hello, where did you get this luetic encephalitis?" "Why do you call it that?" asked the incredulous house physician, Dr. Mosse. Said Sir William: "A completely unilateral paralysis, including face and extremities on the *same* side, in a *young* man who is a sailor (he was widely and visibly tatooed) is most likely due to lues," and so it was!

On another Sunday morning as he walked down the ward he noted a chart with a high, septic fever, and inquired the diagnosis. "Sciatica" was the house physician's reply. "Sciatica, and that fever?" remarked Sir William as he turned down the covers, rolled the patient over and demonstrated a previously unnoted loss of the lumbar lordosis, a beginning kyphosis. He then embarked on a detailed exposition of Pott's disease of the spine with paravertebral abscess and pressure irritation of the lumbar nerve roots, producing sciatic pain. He called for X-ray studies and, as he predicted, they disclosed tuberculous destruction of two lumbar vertebrae.

On another occasion a patient with unexplained diarrhea was presented with the casual statement that amoebic dysentery had been ruled out on the basis of negative smears. "And how were the smears made?" "Stools were sent to the laboratory." "That's no good," and he called for a glove, a rectal tube, a slide, and a microscope. In no time at all he had passed the tube, placed a bit of mucus from the end of the tube on the slide and under the microscope. To the great delight of his audience he demonstrated live, motile, amoeba histolytica.

Despite his fantastic medical knowledge, he too "came a cropper" on rare occasions. A young man with a lower midline abdominal tumor, the size of a large grapefruit, was operated upon with the diagnosis of urachal cyst, a diagnosis in which he had concurred after examination and discussion at Sunday rounds. At operation it proved to be solid. A week later the pathologic diagnosis received by the house surgeon, Dr. McDonald, as we were having afternoon tea, read: "Sarcoma, probably of ovarian origin." Without a word, McDonald jumped up and, dragging me with him, ran down the hall into the ward and to the young man's bed, pulled back the covers to find only one testicle in the scrotum. The obvious diagnosis was sarcoma of an undescended testicle.

The next Sunday morning as the facts were being related to Sir William, his face gradually fell in crestfallen silence. When the sad tale was ended, incriminating so sharply both house staff and consultant, his only comment was: "Gentlemen, these cases are sent to keep us in proper diagnostic humility," and he hurriedly went on to the next case. To his great chagrin, as he revealed later, he had failed to observe two of his own well-born aphorisms: "The abdomen extends from the neck to the knee," and "It is the duty of the consultant to do a rectal examination."

He loved children, and rounds usually ended on the pediatric ward. Children would listen for his coming and regret his parting step. A favorite trick was to put a large English penny on the umbilicus of a bedridden youngster with the promise that "if you keep it there until next Sunday, there'll be two." After Sir William's departure a nurse with farseeing compassion would fix the penny in place with adhesive. Another trick of his informality was to tiptoe into the pediatric ward where the head nurse or sister would be seated at her desk, put his hands before her eyes, saying in a gruff voice: "Guess who's here" to the great delight of the youngsters in the ward.

At a garden party at his Oxford home one sunny afternoon, a staid old dowager duchess was standing directly beneath a second-story balcony with an umbrella opened against the hot sun. Sir William was seen to beckon to two small children, disappear into the house and to reappear on the balcony with a pitcher of water, which he emptied on the good lady's umbrella to the squealing, shouting delight of the children but to the utter dismay of the hostess, Lady Osler.

He had a ready wit and an ever-present sense of humor, much given to practical jokes. When two of his young trainees opened an office next to his on Charles Street in Baltimore they returned one day to find a sign on their lawn reading: "These young fellows are novices—come next door."

He was frequently heard to whistle as he walked along the hospital corridors. Once when asked why he whistled, he replied: "I whistle that I may not weep." What a deeply compassionate nature lies hidden in that simple remark!

During his long last illness, extending over several months of pneumonia, pulmonary abscess and empyema, he once said in a humorously pathetic vein: "How I regret I cannot attend my own postmortem. I've watched the case so long it would be most interesting."

His ashes and magnificent library are now housed in the Osler Library at McGill, thus fulfilling a long-cherished hope:

I like to think of my books in an alcove of a fireproof library in some institution that I love; at the back of the alcove an open fireplace and a few easy chairs, and on the mantelpiece an urn with my ashes, through which my astral self could peek at the books I have loved, and enjoy the delight with which kindred souls still in the flesh would handle them.

Some of his many aphorisms reflect the flair of a schoolmaster as well as the heart of a humanist:

Above everything, gentlemen, come to the study of the diagnosis of disease with all the modesty at your command.

Positiveness and dogmatism are inevitable associates of superficial knowledge in medicine.

Care more for the individual patient than for the special features of the disease.

Keep a looking glass in your own heart, and the more carefully you scan your own frailties, the more tender you are for those of your fellow creatures. In Charity we of the medical profession

must live and move and have our being.

Never believe what a patient may tell you to the detriment of another physician—even though you fear it may be true.

If you can't see good in people, see nothing.

Punctuality is the prime essential of a physician—if invariably on time, he will succeed even in the face of professional mediocrity.

A little old-fashioned courtesy which makes a man shrink from wounding the feelings of a brother practitioner leaves no room for envy, hatred, malice, or any uncharitableness.

The motto of each of you as you undertake the examination and treatment of a case should be: put yourself in his place. Realize so far as you can the mental state of the patient, enter into his feelings, scan gently his faults. The kindly word, the cheerful greeting, the sympathetic look —these the patient understands.

A physician may possess the science of Harvey and the art of Sydenham and yet there may be lacking in him those finer qualities of heart and head which count for so much in life . . . While doctors continue to practice medicine with their hearts as well as their heads, so long will there be a heavy balance in their favor in the bank of Heaven.

This, in brief, was the art of medicine as practiced by Osler. Wrote Welch: "He was in the broadest sense a humanist," but he promptly added Osler's own perceptive comments:

The so-called humanists have not enough science, and science sadly lacks the humanities . . . Twin berries on one stem, grievous damage has been done to both in regarding them in any other light than complemental.

Osler the scientific physician was perhaps over-complemented by Osler the humanist. All his writings, all his actions bespeak his intensely humanistic qualities.

A contrasting personality heavily weighted on the scientific side was that of Osler's good friend and long-time medical colleague, William Stewart Halsted. A thumbnail sketch by Harvey Cushing presented at the time of Halsted's death (1922) is without parallel in its apt epitome of the man:

Professor Halsted, one of the most cultivated and regarded by many as the most eminent surgeon of his time, was a man of unique personality, shy, something of a recluse, fastidious in his tastes and in his friendships, an aristocrat in his breeding, scholarly in his habits, the victim for many years of indifferent health. Nevertheless, he was one of the few American surgeons who may be considered to have established a school of surgery, comparable, in a sense, to the school of Billroth in Vienna. He had few of the qualities supposed to accompany what the world regards as a successful surgeon. Over-modest about his work, indifferent to matters of priority, caring little for the gregarious gatherings of medical men, unassuming, having little interest in private practice, he spent his medical life avoiding patients—even students, when this was possible— and, when health permitted, working in clinic and laboratory at the solution of a succession of problems which aroused his interest. Many of his contributions, not only to his craft but to the science of medicine in general, were fundamental in character and of enduring importance.

Directly emanating from these predominantly non-humanistic traits, and from the abundant and valuable free time they provided to follow his own pursuits, were numerous original surgical procedures, expertly developed in the laboratory or tested in the clinic, and his many original scientific treatises[3] which flowed from his pen to win world-wide acclaim. To mention a few: his introduction of rubber gloves into operating room techniques; his concepts of complete hemostasis and of reducing traumatized tissue in the operative wound to a minimum; his discovery of local anesthesia and its application to dentistry and surgery; his operative techniques for hernia; for carcinoma of the breast with skin grafting; for resection of the thyroid with preservation of the parathyroids; of the aseptic resection of the intestine; his results of the open-air treatment of surgical tuberculosis; his treatment without drainage of a suppurating compound comminuted fracture of the ankle joint; his observations on the training of the surgeon.

His presentations were models of lucid style and diction. Witness the following paragraph (1920):

In a delightful discourse on arteriovenous aneurysm Osler takes a swift flight into a vibrant domain of surgery, tracing into and out of the dark ages steps of the few surgeons who blazed the way. Well he knew and loved the crystal springs and sources bearing their tiny freights of knowledge to the flood. Readers of the Johns Hopkins Hospital Reports will welcome the following quotation from Sir William's paper:

"Better than any other disease aneurysm illustrates how borderless are the boundaries of medicine and surgery. Here am I talking on the most surgical of all its aspects, while very likely not far away a surgeon is practicing the best possible prevention against internal aneurysm in giving a syphilitic patient an injection of Salvarsan®! Aneurysm has been a medico-chirurgical affection ever since some bungling young 'minutor' first nicked the brachial artery in performing venesection. One of the earliest and most interesting references in literature is to an instance of this kind. Galen was called in consultation by a young and inexperienced surgeon who had opened the artery at the bend of the elbow instead of the vein, and the blood spurted out "clarus, rubens, lucidus et calidus."

It is quite apparent that Halsted labored painstakingly over his writing, weighing carefully vocabulary, construction, and meaning. He sought diligently for perfection in the written word, achieved by many revisions—frequently eight to ten—and by consulting ever so diligently his muchthumbed *Century* dictionary.

A letter to Fielding Garrison (dated November 27, 1920, less than two years before his death), reveals his striking preoccupation with style[4]:

We heartily welcome your kindly touches and masterful calligraphic strokes. They recall the pleasure I found, a few years ago, in reading in manuscript a long letter of Swinburne caressingly repolished. You may have noticed that in one of the volumes of Henry James' letters there is reproduced, as a sample of his method, a slice of page proof devoutly slaughtered by his fastidious pencil. How interesting it would be to gather for publication some of the piously revised galley proofs of great writers of poetry and prose. Doubtless you know of such a collection. I have in mind its value to me and to medical men plunging feet first into print, blissfully ignorant of the existence of such a thing as the art of expression or helpless in their search for it.

But these beguiling literary and scientific activities, conducted up to three months before his death, were not sufficiently engrossing to forestall another quite unsuspected activity. Wilder Penfield's fascinating disclosures from Osler's diary[6] revealed that at the very time these original and fundamental advances in surgery were being initiated, developed, and described, Halsted by his own admissions was taking large doses of morphia.

Osler's diary as presented by Penfield records the following important items:

The proneness to seclusion, the slight peculiarities, amounting to eccentricities at times, were the only outward traces of the daily battle through which this brave fellow lived for years. When we recommended him as full surgeon to the Hospital in 1890, I believed, and Welch did too, that he was no longer addicted to morphia. He had worked so well and so energetically that it did not seem possible that he could take the drug and do so much.

About six months after the full position (as Professor of Surgery) had been given, I saw him in a severe chill, and this was the first intimation I had that he was still taking morphia. Subsequently I had many talks about it and gained his full confidence. He had never been able to reduce the amount to less than three grains daily; on this he could do his work comfortably and maintain his excellent physical vigor (for he was a very muscular fellow). I do not think that anyone suspected him, not even Welch.

Subsequently, on Jan. 10, 1898, he got the amount down to 1½ grains, and of late years (1912) has possibly got on without it.

However this may be, important additional information was presented later by Welch. While a patient at Johns Hopkins Hospital for fourteen months preceding his death on April 30, 1934, Welch was under the care of a young house officer named David Sprong, now Professor of Urology at the University of California in Los Angeles. In a letter to me dated May 29, 1968, Dr. Sprong recalls the following statement by Welch:

Although it has been widely reported that Hal-sted conquered his addiction, this is not entirely true. *As long as he lived he would occasionally have a relapse and go back on the drug.* He would always go out of town for this and when he returned he would come to me, very contrite and apologetic, to confess. He had an idea that I could tell what he had done. I couldn't, but I let him go on thinking so because I felt it was good for him to have someone to talk it over with.

Dr. Sprong continued:

I do not remember that Dr. Welch mentioned how long these relapses might last, or how often they occurred, but he felt pretty strongly that the facts should be on the record.

Thus, at long last, through Osler's diary as presented by Penfield, and through Welch's reminiscences as disclosed by Sprong, the probable course of events may be reconstructed:

The early period of addiction (1885-1898) characterized at first by heartrending attempts at control including a futile sea voyage with Welch, and two incarcerations at a Rhode Island hospital, from which he emerged presumably, though actually not cured; a shorter period of less demanding addiction (1898-1912); and the last ten years of his life of semicontrolled addiction characterized by occasional lapses from grace.

We may now hope that the controversy which beguiled both friend and foe for over thirty-eight years is resolved.

As Margaret Boise, his long-time anesthetist, so perceptively wrote in 1952 for the Halsted Centenary[1]: "There was the perennial question as to which road the Professor pursued: the courageous and victorious fight against the enemy, or the equally courageous thirty years of fruitful activity with the haunting enemy always at hand."

Miraculously, despite the long duration of the addiction, there was no deterioration of self, of health, or of mentality. In confirmation of this providential course, the following evidence is presented:

Two years before his death there appeared the impressive volume of "The Operative Story of Goitre,"[3] adjudged to be the most complete and most scholarly study of the subject available.

In the same year appeared his valued monograph on "Ligation of the Left Subclavian Artery in its First Portion."[3]

On April 20, 1920, he, with the assistance of Drs. Heuer and Reid, operated successfully for the second time upon Alexander Miller for the excision of a large left subclavian aneurysm, the subclavian artery having been ligated two years previously by him, in its first portion proximal to the aneurysm.

In the academic year of 1921-22, the year of his death, I, as resident surgeon, assisted him on a number of occasions in the conduct of the Friday Noon Surgical Clinics at which he discussed surgical problems in a most lucid manner. I have vivid memories, for example, of his discussion of the healing that follows the ligation of a large artery. Said he to the students: "John B. Murphy, the Chicago surgeon claims that intima adheres to intima. Not so, when an artery is ligated sufficiently tightly to close its lumen, it also closes the vasa vasorum and the tissue included in the ligature dies, to be replaced by fibrous tissue, as proven in the experimental animal." Turning from the students to me, he continued: "Isn't it a pity Murphy died before knowing this?"

A further example of his erudite mind, active throughout these years, is his far-out philosophical point of view expressed in the concluding remarks of his scholarly Harvey Lecture in March 1914, on "The Significance of the Thymus Gland in Grave's Disease"[3]:

I have touched my subject only very lightly at some of the higher points. Hardly enough has been said even to make it clear that an enormous amount of work underlies the facts which we at present possess. It must be evident to everyone, however, that there reigns the greatest confusion on the subject of the function of the glands of internal secretion.

Fortunately, the ardor for research on our globe is not diminished by the conviction that we are laboring in the wake of workers infinite in numbers on countless worlds who have carried their investigations millions of years beyond the stage reached by us, and are rapidly progressing towards an ultimate solution which may never be reached.

Despite the abstruse character of these observations, they illustrate the wide reaches of his restless mind.

In his last years none suspected his continuing addiction, not even his two secretaries nor his intimate friends, Sam Crowe, Mont Reid, and George Heuer.

In the meantime, a second enemy had appeared. In 1919 his gallbladder had been removed for numerous stones, long held responsible for frequent attacks of abdominal pain. Little improvement followed this operation, and in August 1922, while at his mountain home in North Carolina, he again suffered a severe attack of abdominal pain accompanied by jaundice. After many annoying delays, he set out on a three-day journey to Baltimore by wagon, rail, and ambulance. He arrived at Johns Hopkins Hospital delirious, deeply jaundiced, severely dehydrated, and greatly undernourished.

After massive infusions of normal salt solution he became conscious, entirely lucid, and requested an operation by Drs. Heuer and Reid. This disclosed in the common duct a single stone the size and shape of a large olive. For a few days his condition promised well, but alas, a wound infection developed, accompanied by an aphthous stomatitis, repeated bleeding from rarely encountered aphthous ulcerations of the esophagus and stomach, and finally by a lobar pneumonia of the right upper lobe, which ended in death on September 7, 1922.

In reviewing Halsted's enigmatic though fruitful life, one stands in awe and veneration of this unique and solitary figure, beset through long years by a fearful enemy against which his courage and a strong will repeatedly prevailed to build a life of remarkable achievement. His original conceptions embellished in many areas the art and science of surgery. A valuable legacy to his pupils lay in the inspiration of his dedication to thoughtful inquiry, to the pursuit of perfection, and to the scientific search for truth. In the history of surgery, Halsted clearly and uniquely embodied the role of an original and productive thinker, to whom all surgeons the world over are deeply indebted, now, and in the limitless future.

Has there ever been a saga of more poignant miseries, of more dramatic recoveries, of more magnificent triumphs?

This brief and incomplete study of two contrasting personalities should not detract from the great inspiration and influence each provided in his day. How fortunate that two such vital personalities simultaneously left their permanent mark on the great institution they helped to found and develop. Each complemented the other, and each left a thoroughly individualistic but deep impression on his and subsequent generations.

May the light of these two brilliant stars never be dimmed.

REFERENCES

1. Boise, Margaret: Dr. Halsted as an anesthetist knew him. *Surgery, 32*:498, 1952.
2. Cushing, Harvey: *The Life of Sir William Osler.* Oxford, The Clarendon Press, 1925.
3. Halsted, William Stewart: *Surgical Papers.* Baltimore, The Johns Hopkins Press, 1924.
4. Holman, Emile: William Stewart Halsted as revealed in his letters. *Stanford Med Bull, 10*: 137, 1952.
5. Osler, Sir William: *The Old Humanities and the New Science.* Boston, Houghton Mifflin Co., 1920. Also: New York, The Riverside Press, 1920.
6. Penfield, Wilder: Halsted of Johns Hopkins. *JAMA, 210*:2214, 1969.
7. Thom, Helen Hopkins: *Johns Hopkins, A Silhouette.* Baltimore, The Johns Hopkins Press, 1929. Also: London, Oxford University Press, 1929.

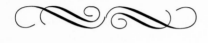

Osler's Opposition To "Whole-Time Clinical Professors"

WILBURT C. DAVISON, M.D.

As a medical student, I saw Sir William Osler frequently during 1913 to 1915, and almost daily as his intern during 1915 to 1916. During that time I heard him say many times that "whole-time clinical professors" would be appointed on the basis of their laboratory and research reputations instead of on their humanistic interest in patients and students, and that research would supplant clinical training and experience. He chuckled in 1913 when he heard that Lewellys F. Barker, the anatomist who succeeded him in 1905 as professor of medicine at The Hopkins, and a one time advocate of "whole time," refused to go on whole-time when the Rockefeller Foundation financed the whole-time clinical program, which Franklin P. Mall, the Hopkins Professor of Anatomy, had been trying to install ever since his original appointment in 1893.

However, it was not until 1960, when Alan M. Chesney,[1] my successor at The Hopkins, gave me a copy of Osler's letter of September 1, 1911, to President Remsen of The Johns Hopkins University,[2] that I realized how bitter Sir William felt, particularly against Abraham Flexner,[3] whom he called "The Angel of Bethesda." I am sure that Osler believed that the appointment of an anatomist with no clinical training or experience as his successor as professor of medicine, was a criticism of his fifteen years at Baltimore. He also probably resented Barker's establishing three laboratories which were concerned primarily with investigation and not with the instruction of students nor with the supervision of patients.

From the following quotations from this 1911 letter, one can readily see his disappointment in his successors at The Hopkins, as well as his sincerity in his beliefs.

Osler pointed out "the falseness of Flexner's statement that the part-time faculty were preventing the complete development of the school, and cited five hundred contributions to scientific medicine from the graduates of the first eight years of The Hopkins which were more brilliant from the clinical than from the laboratory side." He wrote that Flexner's report,[3] "from unfairness or ignorance, was a gross injustice to The Johns Hopkins clinicians."

Osler emphasized that

. . . men whose main interest was the research aspect of medicine and who, like cloistered monks, were out of touch with the rank and file of the medical profession, could not train students for the practice of medicine of which they know nothing and care less.

Do not be led away by the opinions of the pure laboratory men who have no knowledge of the clinical situation or its needs.

And remember what we do today the other schools will try to do tomorrow.

But, lastly and chiefly, divert the ardent laboratory souls who wish to be whole-time clinical professors away from the medical school in which they are not at home to the research institutes to which they properly belong, and in which they can do their best work.

On July 6, 1911, President Remsen wrote Osler that the full-time program suggested by Dr. Mall in 1893 and by Dr. Welch on June 11, 1911, was a *fait accompli*.[1] As a result, Osler's letter of protest to Remsen on September 1, 1911 was ignored, except by Howard A. Kelly, M.D., professor of gynecology, who praised it, and by William H. Howell, Ph.D., professor of physiology, who criticized it.

Osler was not as opposed to "whole-time" as he was to the appointment of laboratory men without clinical experience to teach the practice of medicine. In fact, in his long 1911 letter to Remsen[2] he mentioned "whole-time" only twice. And in his 1919 letter to Magill,[4] he recommended that the clinical professors be "on whole-time or largely so," provided that they were appointed for their clinical ability by a clinical board.

Osler also knew from his own experience as one of the professors of medicine at the University of Pennsylvania from 1884 to 1889 that a laboratory man cannot be a

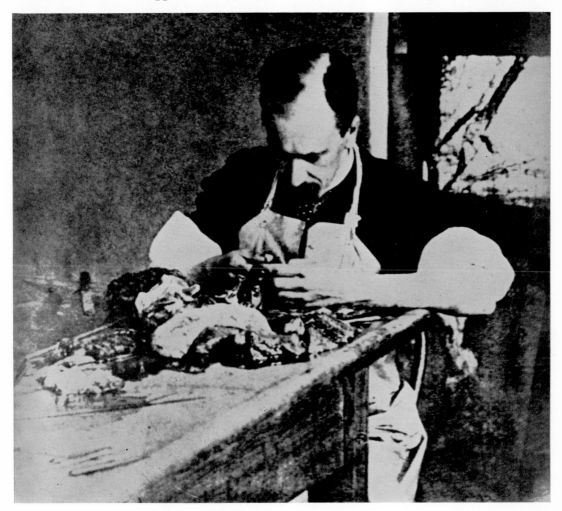

Figure 1. Osler at Old Blockley Hospital—1886.

successful teacher of medical students unless he himself is a good clinician with a humanistic interest in patients and students. When Osler arrived in Philadelphia in 1884 from Montreal he was an excellent pathologist. He knew the end-points of disease but had little experience in the diagnosis and treatment of patients.

Dr. Hezekiah Saiki, whom I met in Kyoto, Japan in 1946, told me that he had been an intern of Osler in Philadelphia from 1885 to 1888. He said that Osler, though he had an office to see private patients, spent most of his time at the Blockley Hospital with students and interns, using his methods of careful history taking, painstaking examination, systematic recording of progress notes, the regular use of the laboratory in the study of the patient, and the introduction of the student into the wards and out-patient department, which later established his reputation and that of The Johns Hopkins Medical School and Hospital.

The results of this work were combined in Osler's immediately famous *Principles and Practice of Medicine* which went through seventeen editions and sold 800,-000 copies, and which provided the income in Baltimore and Oxford which Mall assumed came from private practice.

Mrs. Samuel Gross, the widow of the University of Pennsylvania Medical School Professor of Surgery, told Osler that she would not marry him until the "book" was finished. In 1892, he handed her the book and said: "Now take the man."

One important objection to full time of which Harvey Cushing and Henry Christian warned me in 1927 while organizing the Duke Clinic, but which Osler did not mention in his letter to Remsen because of Mall's mercenary jealousy and antagonism, is that wealthy patients demand to see the head of the clinic. I shall never forget the fury of the wife of the Governor of Pennsylvania, who brought her child to Baltimore on a Saturday afternoon to ask John Howland, the first full-time professor of pediatrics at The Hopkins, whether the child's tonsils should be removed. I examined the child and said, "No." She was not satisfied until she saw Howland on Monday after two days of golf, and he also said "No."

The only private patients Howland would see without protest had rickets or diabetes, but after Edwards Park cured the former with cod liver oil and Sir Frederick Banting cured the latter with insulin, his private practice ceased at the Harriet Lane Home.

As previously mentioned, the "full-time" idea originated with Dr. Franklin P. Mall, the professor of anatomy, when he came to The Hopkins in 1893 as Professor of Anatomy. Dr. Mall had had three years of medical school at Michigan, and a year at a German research institute, but no interest in or knowledge of clinical medicine. Dr. Mall kept up his opposition to Osler until the latter left for Oxford in 1905 with the words: "Mall, now I go, and you have your way." In spite of the glowing story of the life of Dr. Mall by Dr. Florence R. Sabin,[5] Dr. Mall's assistant, many of his colleagues and most of the students found him to be difficult. Finally, in 1907, Dr. Mall persuaded Dr. Welch that the heads of the principal clinical departments, particularly medicine, surgery, pediatrics, and psychiatry, should devote their whole time to teaching and investigation without a busy outside practice.

Fortunately for the students, Dr. Thomas R. Boggs, who had been Resident Physician at The Hopkins since 1909, and who was an inspiring clinical teacher, was appointed Physician-in-Chief of the City Hospital at Bay View and many of the third year Hopkins medical students, even in my time, took their medical quarter there. Dr. Boggs continued Osler's humanistic methods of teaching clinical medicine. He also coached Dr. Barker for his clinics.

Finally on October 21, 1913, Dr. Welch as Chairman of the Administrative Committee of The Hopkins faculty appealed to the General Education Board of the Rockefeller Foundation for funds to implement Dr. Mall's program of whole-time clinical professors. On October 29, 1913, Mr. Wallace Buttrick, the Director of the General Education Board, replied that this request had been granted and that the fund would be called the William H. Welch Endowment for Clinical Education and Research.

The first Hopkins effort to appoint a full-time clinical professor was an invitation to Clemens Freiherr von Pirquet of Vienna to become the professor of pediatrics at a salary of $7,500. However, he demanded $10,000, but funds were insufficient so John Howland was appointed at $4,000. Dr. William S. Halsted became full-time professor of surgery and gave up his private practice. Dr. Lewellys F. Barker, professor of medicine, who originally had been keen on full time, resigned in 1913 because he would not give up his lucrative private practice, and Theodore S. Janeway became the first full-time professor of medicine. Adolf Meyer became the first full-time professor of psychiatry.

These four, though possibly not equal to the original Hopkins "Four Doctors" (Osler, Halsted, Kelly and Welch), painted by Sargent, were excellent clinicians and teachers, so Osler's letters of warning to Remsen[2] and Montreal[4] that "Whole-time Clinical Professors must be Clinicians" were heeded. At any rate, Sir William accepted the invitation to be the principal speaker at the dedication of the Henry Phipps Psy-

chiatric Clinic at The Johns Hopkins on April 16, 1913.

Actually, the first experimental full-time clinical program was at Washington University, St. Louis, with David L. Edsall as professor of medicine, Frederic M. Hanes as assistant professor, and John Howland as professor of pediatrics. It was a flop. Dr. Edsall went to Harvard, Dr. Hanes went into private practice in Winston-Salem, North Carolina, and later became professor of medicine at Duke. As previously stated, Dr. Howland became professor of pediatrics at The Hopkins.

REFERENCES

1. Chesney, Alan M.: *The Johns Hopkins Hospital and The Johns Hopkins University School of Medicine, A Chronicle.* Baltimore, The Johns Hopkins Press, 1963, vols. I, II, and III.
2. Whole-time Clinical Professors—A Letter to President Remsen of The Johns Hopkins University, by William Osler from Oxford, September 1, 1911. This letter was sent to the faculty and trustees of The Hopkins and Mr. Abraham Flexner and marked strictly confidential and not for publication. However, a copy was found among the papers of the late Miss Isabel M. Nutting, Osler's chief nurse, and was published in the *Can Med Assoc J,* 67:762-764, 1962.
3. Flexner, Abraham: Bulletin Number Four, The Carnegie Foundation for the Advancement of Teaching. *Medical Education in the United States and Canada.* 1910.
4. Osler, William: A Circular Letter to Friends in Montreal (Aug. 29, 1919). Sir William Osler Memorial Number, Bulletin IX, International Association of Medical Museums, 1926, pp. 591-2.
5. Sabin, Florence Rena: *Franklin Paine Mall,* Baltimore, The Johns Hopkins Press, 1934; *idem*: The Extension of the Full-time Plan of Teaching in Clinical Medicine, *Science 51:* 1-18, 1922; Fleming, Donald H.: The "full-time" controversy, *The Johns Hopkins Alumni Magazine 6:*11-32, 1954.

Essay V

Osler's Voice

WILDER PENFIELD, M.D.

IT WAS TO THE ART of the practice of medicine that William Osler made his most durable contribution. You may call this art "humanism." But, if you do, let it be understood at once that *humanism in medicine* is something more than the humanism preached, as a gospel, in some other disciplines. If a humanist is to be defined as one who necessarily denies belief in the spirit of man and God, Osler would not have played a willing part in this Galveston symposium. Like Hippocrates, he was not that kind of a humanist. Nor am I, nor some others, I suspect, whom I see gathered here.

The art of the practice of medicine is a spiritual matter and so we would do well to listen to the voice of Osler. He can speak as tellingly today as he did yesterday since we deal with the truth that does not change. Osler was a man who was reticent about his personal beliefs. But he did discuss "Science and Immortality" in his 1904 Ingersoll Lecture at Harvard. He began with the following quotation from the Rubaiyat of Omar Khayyam:

> Strange, is it not? that of the myriads who
> Before us pass'd the door of Darkness through
> No one returns to tell us of the Road,
> Which, to discover, we must travel, too.

Science, Osler explained in the outset, knew nothing about immortality. At the close of his lecture, he answered the question which every man must face by himself, stating simply that to say he believed in it was his own confession of faith. He added the following words, addressed, as usual, to the young men in the audience:

> The hopes and fears which make us men are inseparable, and this wine-press of Doubt each one of you must tread alone. It is a trouble from which no man may deliver his brother or make agreement with another for him. Better that your spirit's bark be driven far from the shore—far from the trembling throng whose sails were never to the tempest given—than that you should tie it up to rot at some lethean wharf.

How did Osler learn to write? And how did he come to be such an excellent clinician? These questions are not directly related to the art of the practice of medicine, to which I have referred. To answer all these questions, we must consider his career. Look with me, then, at the life of this outstanding clinician-scholar. Consider the over-all strategy in distant perspective.

For the first ten years (1874-1884), he was Professor of Medicine at McGill University. During this period, he made his approach to clinical medicine by intensive work in the field of basic science, doing more than a thousand autopsies with his own hand and recording, cataloguing and applying the knowledge gained to the patients in his care. He introduced pathological and physiological methods into his teaching.

During the subsequent five years (1884-1889), as Professor of Medicine at the University of Pennsylvania, he continued to make this scientific approach to clinical medicine, still working at pathology. He crystallized what he had learned and made ready to write his textbook of medicine. This he did during the first two years after his transfer to the Chair of Medicine at the newly-established Medical School of Johns Hopkins. The textbook was a worldwide success in the field of medical practice. But the most important effect of the fifteen years he had spent applying science to practice was what it did to the man who was doing the work. What a practicing-physician it made of him!

In the next sixteen years (1889-1905), he was leader in the field of internal medicine at Johns Hopkins. He introduced teaching at the bedside there and pointed out that it was time for an end to traditional therapy, replacing it with exact analysis, preparing the way for the introduction of specific therapy then in the making on many a laboratory bench.

In the final fourteen years of relative retirement (1905-1919), he turned away from practice and gave more time to books and literature, thus continuing, not beginning, his second career. During this time, his major employment seemed to be what one might call paramedical authorship. This included the essays and addresses related to the human aspects of the lives of physicians and patients, and to the personal problems of the student—medical humanism, no doubt. Through all this time, in all these periods, he enriched the art of the practice of medicine by example as well as precept. The paramedical writings continue to be read today while his textbooks are being placed more and more on the shelves of the medical past.

He stated, when he left Baltimore, that a man produced his best work before forty and added the bitter opinion that little could be expected after the age of sixty. That generalization is open to question now, particularly because of the evidence provided in his own life. Cushing's excellent account of the Osler epic—the forty-five years as professor of medicine that came to an end when he died in 1919—resulted in two large volumes. The whole of the second

volume is required to tell what Cushing thought to be important during the Oxford period! These were the twilight years of a medical man and yet who shall say that the output was of less value to the world than all that went before?

And now, since I am one of the hardy perennials who knew him in student days, let me talk of the man who led this life, and may the good Lord help us to understand how he did what he did. William Osler, when I knew him, was a spare, swarthy, quick-moving man with an oft-returning twinkle in his brown eyes. He must have resembled his mother, an indomitable little woman with the olive complexion that betrayed her descent from the ancient Celts of Cornwall. His father was an adventurous gray-eyed Anglo-Saxon who came to Bond Head, Upper Canada, to propagate "the gospel in foreign parts." His father intended Willie for the Church. Toward that end, Willie received a standard classical education. Late in his career, he told the story of what might be called his conversion to the microscope. This, oddly enough, was printed in *The School World,* a London publication, in 1916. In addition to the conversion, it explained his escape from the classics, as presented to him in Greek and Latin, as well as how he rediscovered the classics in translation.

Ten years with really able . . . teachers, left me with no more real knowledge of Greek and Latin than of Chinese, and without the free use of the language as keys to great literature. Imagine the delight of a boy of an inquisitive nature to meet a man (W. A. Johnson*) who cared nothing about words but who knew about things —who knew the stars in their courses and who could tell us their names, who delighted in the woods in springtime, and told us about the frogspawn and the caddis worms, and who read to us in the evenings . . . who showed us with the microscope the marvels in a drop of dirty pond

*"Father Johnson" was founder of the Weston School which later became Trinity College School of Port Hope.

water, and who on Saturday excursions up the river could talk of the Trilobites and Orthoceratites and explain the formation of the earth's crust. No more dry husks for me after such a diet . . . From the study of nature to the study of man was an easy step.

To step from "the study of nature to the study of man" seemed easy to him in retrospect. But how did the growing boy and the maturing man do it? The answer calls for a full length biography. Cushing carried out his assigned task of assembling the material and did it well. Edith Gittings Reid, in _The Great Physician,_* has given us what is, in my opinion, the clearest glimpse of the man. But it is incomplete. She had loved him as a little child when he used to appear in her parents' New York home and come running up the stairs to her nursery, a man with long moustaches and twinkling eyes, as full of Puckish glee and fancy as any child. When she grew older, she understood him as only a woman can, perhaps. But the biography that will tell the inner story of this physician waits for its author.

How can I help you to know this simple, unpretentious man? How make you see him with his high forehead and the impassive face, the twinkle, the quick smile, the ready laugh? How can I cause you to hear him saying good-by to an anxious student, opening the door, reassuring him with few words, approving his plan of life and sending him off on his bicycle through the rain with renewed courage and the warm awareness that he has a friend?

I was that medical student. Two other American Rhodes Scholars were medical students at Oxford with me, Emile Holman and Wilburt Davison. The Englishmen and the Scots who should have been our comrades had gone to serve their country in the First World War, and some, alas, to die.

*Edith Gittings Reid: _The Great Physician._ Oxford, Oxford University Press, 1931.

We three left Oxford in 1916, a year before the United States joined the conflict, entering Johns Hopkins Medical School.

In 1919, I went back to Oxford, this time as a graduate student in physiology. I arrived during Sir William's last illness and, when they bore him from Norham Gardens to Christ Church Cathedral, I followed and sat alone at the back. Someone at the lectern high above us said that the man who was dead had been "a friend of all young men." And so he had. I thought then I was losing him but, strange to say, it was not so. Even today that "warm awareness" that I have a friend lingers on. Isn't that, after all, a happy sort of immortality for him?

It was Fielding H. Garrison who wrote the tribute I like to quote. He called himself a pupil of Osler, and he was a medical historian with a total perspective of the story of our profession.

We shall scarcely look upon his like again . . . What Osler meant to the medical profession in America, what he did for us, can never be adequately expressed . . . He was handsome, wise, witty, learned, courteous, fair-minded and brave . . . a bond between English-speaking physicians everywhere.

In 1913, Osler, at the age of sixty-four, accepted the invitation of Yale University to give the Silliman Lectures on _The Evolution of Modern Medicine._ He returned from Oxford to New Haven and while there he was called upon to address the Yale students on a Sunday evening. It was then that he talked about _how_ he had done what he did in medicine. The address was called _A Way of Life_ and was published then.

It is interesting that Osler, himself, never did finish the preparation of the lectures on _The Evolution of Modern Medicine_ even during the six years that remained to him after their delivery. They were finished for him after his death and published in 1921 by the Yale Press. If the history of medicine had been his major concern during the Oxford years, he would have put this project first and finished it with enthusiasm. Instead of doing that, he was fully occupied by his concern for the art of the practice of medicine and fascinated by the writings of others, even through the years of the 1914 to 1918 war.

Six years after these lectures at Yale—it was the last year of his life—Osler went up to London on a consultation and happened on a poem that expressed, he thought, the message he meant to leave with the Yale students. The patient he had come to see was a remarkable woman, under sentence of death from cancer. She had translated the poem from the Sanskrit herself and had woven it into an old-fashioned sampler in which Osler discovered it. Here is the poem,* in part:

> Listen to the Exhortation of the Dawn!
> Look to this Day! . . .
> For yesterday is but a Dream
> And Tomorrow is only a Vision;
> But To-day, well lived, makes
> Every Yesterday a Dream of Happiness,
> And every Tomorrow a Vision of Hope.
> Look well therefore to this Day!
> Such is the Salutation of the Dawn!

The way of life that Osler preached was simple and simply expressed. Our main business, he said, was "to do what lies clearly at hand!" Learn to concentrate at your work a few hours each day and give a few minutes to better reading so that you may have "fellowship with the great minds of the race."

He talked of the gospel of work. But this was a gospel he expressed even better, according to my way of thinking, ten years before when he was addressing the undergraduates of the University of Toronto.

*The author of this poem, William Francis told me, is an Indian dramatist who lived about 400 AD, Kalidasa by name. The poem was added, according to Osler's wish, to the second edition of the lecture, published in New York and London by Harper Brothers in 1937.

That earlier talk was called *The Master Word in Medicine*.† The master word was "work." "It is," he wrote, "the open sesame to every portal, the great equalizer in the world, the true philosopher's stone, which transmutes all the base metal of humanity into gold. The stupid man among you it will make bright, the bright man brilliant and the brilliant student steady."

There is much beautiful writing like that in *The Master Word*. It makes one realize that Osler had a fault, a serious defect. Now don't rise up in protest and leave your seats. The truth is that he overloaded some of his addresses with quotations. They sparkled, one after the other, like a succession of exotic gems until the dazzled reader longed to return to the simple superiority of Osler's own thinking and writing.

No one is so apt to tell a man his defects, and likewise recognize his virtues, as an intelligent and understanding wife. Lady Osler was all of that as well as a woman of generous charm and intuition. But unfortunately, perhaps for William Osler, she was otherwise occupied with Dr. William Gross, a surgeon of Philadelphia, until the death of Gross just as Osler was leaving Philadelphia for Baltimore. Osler returned to marry Mrs. Gross, the former Grace Revere, when he was forty-three, having finished his book. No doubt he was less plastic than he would have been twenty years earlier when he was beginning to develop his skill in speaking and writing. In any case, long after the wedding day, when the Oslers took me into their home for a fortnight's convalescence, their union seemed to me the happiest of marriages and she was clearly the critic he turned to for the criticism that every writer needs.

After I had given as the title of this ad-

†William Osler: *Aequanimitas*. London, Lewis, 1914.

dress, *Osler's Voice,* I realized how presumptuous it was of me. I went to the Osler Library at McGill one evening in a mood of desperation. Donald Bates, Ellen Wells, Edward Bensley and the others who bring that library to life each morning were safe at home. I sat and pondered, quite alone. What should I say to those who would be gathered in Galveston? Your splendid tribute to the man, fifty years after his spirit passed out through the "door of Darkness," called for something beyond the commonplace.

Around me, from floor to ceiling, there were shelves of books. You know, of course, that after his death in Oxford, Osler's books were catalogued and brought to McGill University by his nephew, William Francis, in accordance with Sir William's will and Lady Osler's anxious prodding. The central room of the library is elegant and friendly. It seemed to me to be filled with thoughts —thoughts from the past and the thinking of the present, thoughts of the great physicians of long ago and of Osler, Francis, Cécile Desbarats and memories of Archibald Malloch and Harvey Cushing. Thoughts do live on,* you know, and intermingle with all that is contemporary. And this is another sort of happy immortality for Osler.

The walls of the room, as I have said, are lined with books from ceiling to floor except that, at the far end, there is a panel of polished wood. Behind that panel, which bears no name, the ashes of Sir William and his lady rest, hidden away according to their request. What could I say, I wondered. What would please him and interest you who are already his intimate friends? Some of you are distinguished historians, highly critical scholars.

---

*Chauncey D. Leake amplified this idea beautifully by a spontaneous poem, "thoughts do live on," written during the meeting.

Impulsively, I turned toward the panel and spoke aloud: "Sir William, won't you come along with me?" The room was in shadow except for the circle of light on the table before me. I picked up two notebooks that had been left there at my request. In them, as a school boy, Willie Osler had copied out his Greek verbs. On the fly leaf, he had written very uncomplimentary opinions of certain school fellows. Then, in another hand, there was the pencilled observation, "Osler, you are a perfect goose!"

I chuckled out loud and, as I did so, I heard a sound behind me. Was it a laugh? or only the wind shaking the windows? I turned quickly. No. And no one had entered.

I was glad to be alone. So I sat down and began to think things over. Indeed, I may have grown a little sleepy. I often do when I've nothing more stimulating than my own thoughts.

Young Osler, I mused, was just a boy like other boys, a mixture of good and bad to begin with. Even though he was the head of his form at Trinity College School, it seems that he was far from perfect in the outset. Later in life, of course, he developed many talents and he was a master of polished phrase, but his early addresses were stilted, halting, *gauche.* I know, for I have made a careful comparative study.

Feeling myself alone there in the library, and yet in such good company, I began to speak out loud. "How," I exclaimed, "did you grow up to be the man the world knew? I wonder if other boys in your form could not have done just as well as you did, if they had used your formula of life and work and play."

There was a crash in the silent room! And I leaped from my chair. A book had fallen from a high shelf to the floor. That was strange. A tingling sensation began in the top of my head and spread down my spine. Cool air, it seemed to me, was moving as though a door had been opened. I looked down at the book. It lay open on the floor. The leaves fluttered just a little. I walked into the alcove, making as much noise as possible and clearing my throat. Nothing there except Billie Francis's desk. It had been Sir William's. I had known it as his when a blessed broken-leg made me a guest in their home. That was so long ago. No one in the other alcove. The storm outside did seem to be shaking the windows. I picked up the book.

It was open to an address—the one Osler gave to the undergraduates at Yale on *A Way of Life*. Not his best bit of writing, but the one in which he really talked about himself, told of his life in four universities, professor in all four. I began to read.

A man who has filled Chairs in four universities, has written a successful book and has been asked to lecture at Yale, is supposed, popularly, to have brains of a special quality. A few of my intimate friends really know the truth about me, as I know it! Mine, in good faith I say it, are of the most mediocre character.

Those were Osler's own words. Unconsciously, I looked toward the panel at the end of the room and spoke aloud. "What about those four professorships?" I said. "How did they happen to come to you?" There was no movement but I seemed to hear a voice, these words: "Just a habit, a way of life, an outcome of the day's work . . ." Osler's voice had repeated those words! I heard it, and yet the words were printed, on the page before me!

Phantom hair was standing up all along my back and even on the top of my head where there has been no proper hair, alas, for far too long a time.

Then, again, I heard the voice. It *was* Osler's voice. How well I knew it! Once, in 1916, I had listened in his own library

at 13 Norham Gardens while he read, sitting at his desk, the address he was to make at the Bodleian Library on the following day, while Lady Osler and their son, Revere, made comments and, at the end, she gave her words of approbation. Now, in the silence of his McGill Library, he seemed to be speaking quietly, as he had in Oxford. He never had an accent that one could identify. Really-good speakers, I have noticed (like the Southerner, Woodrow Wilson, and the man from Buckingham Palace, George the Sixth) manage to speak an English that is pure and almost free of accent. Osler spoke as I have heard them speak.

The voice was continuing:

As I look back each new phase in my growing-up came naturally because of my way of life. It was all the outcome of the day's work. Nothing complicated. I started the day with a private prayer. I ended the day reading good literature for 15 to 20 minutes and I made notes on the books I read. I worked hard at the daily job and loved it. I suppose I was looking always for something better. Curiously enough it was the minor incidents that seemed to shape my life. Take for instance how I happened to go to Trinity School. Read about it in the book before you.

So, I read aloud as follows:

I was diverted to Trinity College School, then at Weston, Ontario, by a paragraph in the circular stating that the senior boys would go into the drawing room in the evenings, and learn to sing and dance—vocal and pedal accomplishments for which I was never designed; but, like Saul seeking his asses, I found something more valuable—a man who knew nature, and who knew how to get boys interested in it.

I looked up from the book, half expecting to see Osler laughing at me. But no, I was alone. Then I seemed to hear his voice again. "I'm nearly always present," he said, "one way or another, when men talk of how to practice medicine. They call on me to speak again even now after fifty years!"

I had a feeling of fear then and wondered vaguely if I could be dreaming. But now, as I look back, I realize it was all quite different from a dream. When I was writing out what is written in this manuscript, I was frightened and my heart did pound. Those are facts, not fancies.

At last, I seemed to hear Sir William sigh, quite close to me. I waited in breathless silence:

It is good to live on with all of you on the other side of the door. Immortality comes in ways you may not understand. The spirit must be prepared for it before you pass the door of darkness—just a habit, a way of life, and work. Work, thus "transmutes the base metal of humanity into gold."

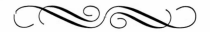

Essay VI

The Men Who Inspired William Osler[*]

R. PALMER HOWARD, M.D.

A RECENT READING of Osler's essays and biographical writings led me to the question—who stimulated Osler? Cushing closed the *Life* with an arresting portrayal of the burial service at Christ Church Chapel. Browne's *Religio Medici* lay on the coffin and Robert Burton's statue was nearby. The heart-wringing final paragraph reads in part:

> And perhaps that New Year night saw, led by Revere, another procession pass by the 'watching-chamber'—the spirits of many, old and young—of former and modern times—of Linacre, Harvey, and Sydenham; of John Locke, Gesner, and Louis; of Bartlett, Beaumont, and Bassett; of Johnson, Bovell, and Howard; of Mitchell, Leidy and Stillé; of Gilman, Billings, and Trudeau; of Hutchinson, Horsley, and Payne; of the younger men his pupils who had gone before . . .[1]

Osler as youth or man responded warmly to all manner and ages of people. He coupled a sympathetic interest in the lives of the authors with his wide perusal of medical, scientific, and literary works. Even

during his crowded professional life, Osler spared at least half an hour every day for reading the world's great literature. It is not easy to select from the many who inspired him. Osler's own writings have been the chief resource, but articles by Brush,[2] Welch,[3] Keynes,[4] and others, have been helpful.

The ninth child of a Cornish missionary on the Canadian frontier, William was nurtured on the King James Bible. From this he drew much of his writing style and many quotations. His bonds were always close with his parents and every member of his family. William proceeded along the course of parental desire to become a clergyman. In preparation he attended Trinity College School at Weston, Ontario. Osler boarded with the warden, the Reverend William A. Johnson. This devout Anglican priest was also an ardent naturalist who led the boys to pond, field and cave. He stimulated them to mount and study their treasures under the microscope.

Johnson also helped shape Osler's general cultural development. While still a schoolboy, he acquired a one-volume Shakespeare and a recent edition of Sir Thomas Browne's *Religio Medici* (1642). Both books influenced Osler deeply. Browne's philosophy, a blending of unbridled curiosity and scholarly contemplation about na-

*From Howard, R. Palmer: The men who inspired Osler. *South Med J, 65*: 232-235, 1972.

ture and mankind with a firm but simple Christian faith, became Osler's support along the road of life.

"Father" Johnson and his friend, Dr. James Bovell, unwittingly led Osler to change from divinity to medicine in 1865 after his first year at Trinity College, Toronto. Dr. Bovell was a man of many sides, too diffuse to accomplish his goals. Yet he stimulated his young pupil to learn microscopic and other laboratory methods and, at the same time, influenced Osler to read widely among the great books of science and literature. The life of Bovell served in many ways as a warning rather than a model. Bovell lacked organization and punctuality. He dissipated his energies in attempts to interpret the mysteries of life from scientific and religious aspects at the same time. Though Osler avoided these pitfalls, Bovell's influence, nevertheless, was powerful and enduring.[5,6]

In 1870, when Bovell left Toronto for the West Indies, Osler followed his advice and transferred to the McGill Medical School because of better clinical facilities in Montreal. The senior physician at the Montreal General Hospital, Robert Palmer Howard (1823-1889), soon became Osler's patron, prompter, fellow-student, and friend. In his house was the largest and most up-to-date collection of medical books in Montreal, and this library was freely available to the young student. In addition, Howard was interested in pathology, and performed thorough autopsies on his own cases. Osler's ability in microscopic techniques was quickly recognized, and Howard demonstrated his student's preparations at medical meetings. Mutual friendship and respect led to strong and lifelong bonds.

The McGill clinicians by tradition followed Edinburgh's clinical teaching methods, which pupils of Boerhaave carried there from Leyden. After graduating from McGill, Howard studied with the great Dublin clinicians, Graves and Stokes, whose inspiration came from the Paris of Laennec and Louis. In his long career of medical practice and student teaching at the Montreal General Hospital, Howard endeavored to keep up with the clinical and laboratory advances from Germany and France. When Osler was a senior student in 1871, Howard insisted that all patients suspected of pulmonary tuberculosis be shown him for review and comparison with pathological specimens. Howard was Professor of Medicine and later Dean of the McGill Medical School, a leader of his profession throughout Canada, and a respected confrere of the American medical professors.[8-11] Osler dedicated *The Principles and Practice of Medicine* (1892) to Johnson, Bovell, and Howard.

Rudolf Virchow's (1821-1902) influence began when Osler was a student in Berlin in 1873. On his return from Europe, Osler taught physiology and pathology while Professor of the Institutes of Medicine at McGill. He continued this interest at the Blockley Hospital in Philadelphia and at Johns Hopkins. Along these lines Osler stimulated many students, including Maude Abbott who developed a pathological museum and wrote a classical account of congenital heart disease. Osler's address in honor of Virchow is ample evidence of the influence exerted by "the greatest pathologist since John Hunter."[12] One of his first purchases in Montreal was Virchow's handbook, and this volume found a treasured place among Virchow's other books in the *B. Prima* of the *Bibliotheca Osleriana*.[13]

Henceforth my theme follows a threefold course; Linacre, Harvey and Sydenham— letters, science, and practice. As a young medical graduate in 1873, Osler fell under the influence of the English clinicians as well as the libraries in London and elsewhere. The panel painting of the three great Englishmen typifies Osler's own career, though he did not see it until 1894, when he visited Sir Henry Acland, the Regius Professor at Oxford. Osler's wife Grace persuaded Acland to have a copy made to place over their mantle in Baltimore, little knowing that Osler would fall academic heir to the original panel when he, too, became Regius Professor at Oxford in 1905.[14,15]

Thomas Linacre (1460-1524) a principal founder of the College of Physicians of London, was a hero and model for Osler from his early years.[16,17] Linacre is best known for translating many of Galen's books from Greek into Latin prose of unparalleled grace, and being the teacher of Erasmus. As Welch remarked in discussing Osler's presidential address "Old Humanities and New Sciences,"[18] Linacre was the only physician before Osler with qualifications appropriate for election as president of the Classical Association.[19]

William Harvey (1578-1657) was the greatest scientist to appear among the English physicians. A Cambridge graduate and a follower of John Caius, he learned the existence of the venous valves and drew his inspiration from Fabricius at Padua. Harvey's quantitative experimental study of the circulation laid the foundation for the science of physiology. Osler's Harveian Oration illustrated his appreciation.[20]

Thomas Sydenham (1624-1689) made important contributions to the knowledge of acute fevers and gout, but was best known as the model practitioner of his age, the English Hippocrates.[16] Osler's interest in Sydenham was apparently reinforced by John Brown's biographical essays.[21,22]

From the literary influence of Shake-speare, Thomas Browne, and Linacre, may be derived a long series of writers, ancient and contemporary, whom Osler respected and emulated. Early in his career he became an ardent disciple of Plato, whom he quoted frequently in his addresses.[23,24] The high place of Thomas Browne in Osler's estimation as "the most liberal of men and most distinguished of general practitioners" is a recurrent theme in his writings and remarks.[25-27] Osler's analysis of the creators, transmuters and transmitters of knowledge revealed his devotion to Shakespeare and Robert Burton, as well as his respect for the contributions of the transmuters, such as Francis Bacon.[28] The bonds with Robert Burton, the Oxford cleric and author of *The Anatomy of Melancholy,* were particularly strong. Osler credited the survival of this work to Burton's human sympathy.[29] Osler, the physician, though often gay, was also deeply moved by the phenomena of death.[30] Some of his later English friends, indeed, interpreted Osler's underlying personality as one of melancholy, at least in the sense of a deep sensitivity to the inescapable sadness of humanity.[31]

Several prominent nineteenth century medical men who owed their reputations in large measure to their literary skills, also influenced Osler. Oliver Wendell Holmes, who taught anatomy at Harvard and promulgated the contagiousness of puerperal fever, wrote "The Autocrat of the Breakfast Table" and "The Chambered Nautilus."[32] John Brown, physician of Edinburgh, included "Rab and His Friends," with essays on Locke, Sydenham, and Dr. Francis Adams of Banchory.[33] Elisha Bartlett, the Rhode Island native, wrote clearly on the epidemic fevers and other professional matters, and also an imaginative essay on Hippocrates.[34] S. Weir Mitchell gained fame from his original writings in neurology and also from his poetry. Mitchell was one of Osler's sponsors for the appointment at Philadelphia, and they remained lifelong friends.[35]

Osler's interest in John Locke may have sprung from his admiration of Thomas Sydenham, Locke's preceptor and friend. Osler explored Locke's medical writings and practice before and during his appointment as physician to Ashley Cooper, the founder of Carolina Colony.[36] Locke's works include the *Epistle on Toleration,* the *Constitution of Carolina,* and *An Essay Concerning Humane Understanding.* The originality and enduring vitality of his philosophical works, rather than his contributions to clinical medicine, account for Locke's place in the *prima* section of the *Bibliotheca Osleriana.*

John Keats, the physician-poet, Percy Bysshe Shelley, Ralph Waldo Emerson, and Walt Whitman influenced Osler through their skills in interpreting the sensitivity of the human spirit. Perhaps I should also include John Newman, the Oxford religious philosopher who later became Cardinal. A revered English aunt gave Osler Newman's portrait, which held a prominent place in his study.[37]

Three other men are best classified with the literary group. Osler's interest arose largely because of their achievements in bibliography and librarianship, although each was also prominent in other fields of medicine. Important among these was Conrad Gesner (1516-1565), the father of bibliography, whose place in the *B. Prima* is explained in the editors' preface and the footnote in the *Bibliotheca Osleriana.*[38-39] W. H. Welch interpreted Osler's admiration for Gesner as a reflection of the many noble attributes they held in common.[40]

John Shaw Billings (1838-1913), the chief builder and bibliographer of the Surgeon General's Library, was also a leading figure in the planning of the Johns Hopkins Hospital. To Billings fell the task of inviting Osler to head the Department of Medicine in 1889. Osler admired his talents as librarian, historian, sanitationist and administrator. Osler's recognition of his important contributions, as well as their long cordial acquaintance, testify to Billings' influence on his younger colleague.[41,42] Joseph F. Payne (1840-1910) shared with Osler an interest in history, an appreciation of Harvey and Sydenham, and an eager love for book collecting. The older Payne may have stimulated Osler's bibliophilic and bibliographic endeavors during a visit in 1899. Osler eulogized his friend as an outstanding British medical scholar.[43,44]

In addition to Harvey and Virchow, medical scientists influential on Osler included the physiologist, John Burdon Sanderson (1828-1905). In the latter's laboratory, Osler studied the platelets in the circulating blood in 1874.[45] Osler wrote admiring sketches on the lives of the great French chemist - microbiologist Louis Pasteur (1822-1895),[46] and the American "backwoods physiologist" William Beaumont (1785-1853).[47] The American military surgeon's patient, Alexis St. Martin, was buried near Montreal without loss of the fistulous stomach to Osler's designs for its preservation in the museum of the United States Army Surgeon General.[48,49]

Among his own American colleagues, two other physician-scientists made deep impressions on Osler. Joseph Leidy (1823-1891), the outstanding American contributor to paleontology and parasitology, was still active in the biological societies and academic circles of Philadelphia during Osler's sojourn in that city. Although he commented that Leidy lacked Charles Darwin's power to derive general laws from his far-reaching observations, Osler's remarks in

"The Leaven of Science" remain a lasting tribute.[50]

It is difficult to evaluate the importance of William H. Welch (1850-1934) on Osler's clinical and historical writings. Welch was the senior in time of appointment among the "Big Four" at Hopkins, and became the leader of scientific medicine in Baltimore and the American continent. Osler appreciated his excellence in scientific demonstration and publication, judgment in selecting other professors, skill in training young men, and the collaboration with the studies of the vigorous young clinical investigators. Welch, Billings and Osler founded the Historical Club at the Johns Hopkins Medical School. Osler always respected Welch deeply as an administrator and planner in education. Though on opposing sides in the controversy over full time clinical teaching in the decade before the World War, Osler and Welch remained warm friends, as Osler's writings amply testify.[51,52]

Many other followers of Sydenham strongly influenced "The Great Physician" of this century. Osler, of course, included René Laennec (1787-1826) in his *B. Prima* and referred to him frequently in his writings. Since his early associations with the McGill professors, Osler held the highest regard for the man upon whom Laennec's mantle fell, Pierre Charles Alexandre Louis (1787-1872). Osler recognized Louis' great influence on American medicine through his statistical evaluation of clinical treatment and his reports on epidemic fevers, tuberculosis, and bloodletting. More important was the long line of distinguished Americans trained in part by the other Parisian contemporaries, but especially by Louis.[53,54] With reference to this influence on American physicians Osler quoted from Oliver Wendell Holmes on the three lessons

brought from Paris: "not to take authority when I can have facts, not to guess when I can know, and not to think a man must take physic because he is sick."[55] These, indeed, were characteristics of Osler's own medical practice.

Another of Louis' pupils, Alfred Stillé (1813-1900), was Osler's predecessor as professor of medicine at Philadelphia. He wrote the first American book on general pathology, the encyclopedic *National Dispensatory* (1879),[56] and an important paper on epidemic meningitis. The clue to Osler's admiration of this elder statesman of American medicine is given by the concluding quotation from Stillé: "Only two things are essential, to live uprightly and to be wisely industrious."[57] Osler followed both precepts.

Well known, also, is Osler's tribute to another American visitor to Paris, John Y. Bassett, the dedicated practitioner in the Alabama countryside, and studious observer of the local epidemics. In "An Alabama Student" Osler not only honored his fellow-physicians on the front line, but revealed a motivating influence behind his own method of teaching clinical medicine.[58]

Osler's Oxford house contained a portrait of Horatio C. Wood of Philadelphia (1841-1920). Wood visited Montreal as chairman of the Selection Committee in 1884. Osler admired his contributions to biology and clinical medicine, and they maintained an active correspondence.[59,60] Important, also, were several prominent British clinicians, such as Henry Acland, Clifford Albutt, Jonathan Hutchinson, Victor Horsley and Humphrey Rolleston, and the young historian Charles Singer. Osler admired men like these wherever he encountered them. Surely such friendships led to mutual stimulation.

Finally, reference must be made to one

who was not a practicing physician, but an educational administrator. President Daniel Coit Gilman formulated the program and assembled the faculty for the Johns Hopkins University, and later effected the opening of the hospital by serving as its first superintendent.[61] Clearly, Gilman played a dominant role in guiding the development of the separate but coordinated institutions. Osler always held him in high esteem. In 1904 he dedicated *Aequanimitas With Other Addresses* to Gilman in words ending: "In grateful recognition of your active and intelligent interest in medical education."[62]

Were some influences on Osler more important than others? Shakespeare and Thomas Browne yield place to none. Let us turn once more, however, to two of Harvey Cushing's triads of spirits by the "watching-chamber"—Johnson, Bovell and Howard; and Linacre, Harvey and Sydenham. The inspiration Osler drew from the parson-naturalist Johnson and the practitioner-clinical professor Howard outlasted that from the biologist-physician Bovell. The greats from olden times provide a parallelism. Osler obtained a thorough grounding in the laboratory sciences, appreciated the significance of new discoveries and, furthermore, stimulated his students towards investigative work. He gave the first place of honor to William Harvey and other contributors of original ideas, but with an apt self-evaluation he concentrated his own efforts chiefly on the literary and medical practice spheres of his famous heroes, Linacre and Sydenham.

While a young professor on the wards at McGill, Osler brought new life to the clinical teaching of Boerhaave, the Scottish and Irish clinicians, and their Canadian followers. He advanced the system in Philadelphia and developed it to fruition in the undergraduate teaching and the medical residency program of the Johns Hopkins Medical School. Yet, in Canada, the United States and England, he also stimulated his fellow-physicians and students to read medical books and journals, and the classics of the world's literature. Neophytes in the profession were led to draw inspiration from the appreciation of human values expressed by the great men of the past, and to follow these guideposts throughout their lives. Osler taught students on the wards but, even more importantly, through his interpretation of history and by his own acts as physician, colleague and friend, he showed all men the "way of life."

REFERENCES

1. Cushing, H.: *The Life of Sir William Osler.* Oxford, Clarendon Press, vol. 2, p. 686, 1925.
2. Brush, E. N.: Osler's literary style. *Bull Hopkins Hosp, 30:*217-233, 1919.
3. Welch, W. H.: Foreword. In Abbott, M. E. (ed): *Sir William Osler Memorial Volume. Bulletin No. 9, International Association of Medical Museums,* Montreal, pp. *i-xi,* 1926.
4. Keynes, G.: The Oslerian tradition. *Brit Med J, 4:*599-604, 1968.
5. Osler, W.: The master-word in medicine. In *Aequanimitas With Other Addresses to Medical Students, Nurses and Practitioners of Medicine.* Philadelphia, Blakiston Co., pp. 369-371, 1904; 3rd ed. pp. 353-355, 1932.
6. Dolman, C. E.: The Reverend James Bovell, M.D., 1817-1888. *In Pioneers of Canadian Science; Royal Society of Canada,* Toronto: Univ of Toronto Press, pp. 81-100, 1966.
7. Osler, W.: An address on the medical clinic; a retrospect and a forecast. *Brit Med J, 1:*10-16, 1914.
8. _____ The student life. In *Aequanimitas,* 3rd ed. pp. 420-421, 1932.
9. Howard, R. P.: Introductory address: a sketch of the life of the late Dr. G. W. Campbell, and a summary of the early history of the faculty. In *Medical Faculty, McGill College Semi-Centennial Celebration,* Montreal pp. 1-24, 1882.

10. Osler, W.: Robert Palmer Howard, M.D. *Med News, 54*:419, 1889.
11. Cushing, H.: *Life,* vol. 1, pp. 83-85, 131.
12. Osler, W.: Rudolf Virchow: The man and the student. *Boston Med Surg J, 125*:425-427, 1891.
13. _____*Bibliotheca Osleriana: A Catalogue of Books Illustrating the History of Medicine and Science, Collected, Arranged and Annotated by Sir William Osler, Bt., and Bequeathed to McGill University.* Oxford, Clarendon Press, pp. *xix,* 158-161, 1929.
14. Cushing, H.: *Life,* vol. 1, p. 401.
15. Acland, T. D.: The Oxford University Museum. In *Contributions to Medical and Biological Research, Dedicated to Sir William Osler . . . ,* New York, Paul Hoeber, vol. 1, p. 2, 1919.
16. Osler, W.: British medicine in Greater Britain. *Brit Med J, 2*:576-581, 1897.
17. _____ *Thomas Linacre.* Cambridge, Cambridge Univ Press, 1908.
18. _____ The old humanities and the new science. *Brit Med J, 2*:1-7, 1919.
19. Cushing, H.: *Life,* vol. 2, pp. 650-651.
20. Osler, W.: The growth of truth as illustrated in the discovery of the circulation of the blood. *Brit Med J, 2*:1077-1084, 1906.
21. Brown, J.: *Horae Subsecivae. Locke and Sydenham, With Other Occasional Papers.* Edinburgh, 1858.
22. Osler, W.: *Bibliotheca,* No. 4396.
23. Cushing, H.: *Life,* vol. 1, p. 370.
24. Osler, W.: Physic and physicians as depicted in Plato. *Boston Med Surg J, 128*:129-133, 153-156, 1893.
25. _____ Chauvinism in medicine. *Montreal Med J, 31*:684-699, 1902.
26. _____ Sir Thomas Browne. *Brit Med J, 2*:993-998, 1905.
27. Keynes, G.: The Oslerian tradition, pp. 599-600, 604.
28. Osler, W.: *Creators, Transmuters and Transmitters: As Illustrated by Shakespeare, Bacon, and Burton* (remarks at the opening of the Bodley Shakespeare Exhibition, April 24, 1916). London, Oxford Press, 1916.
29. _____ Robert Burton, the man, his book, his library. In *Selected Writings of Sir William Osler . . .,* London, Oxford Univ Press, pp. 65-99, 1951.
30. _____*Science and Immortality.* Boston, Houghton, Mifflin & Co., 1904.
31. Bett, W. R.: *Osler, The Man and The Legend.* London, William Heinemann Medical Books, Ltd., p. 118, 1951.
32. Osler, W.: Oliver Wendell Holmes. *Bull Hopkins Hosp, 5*:85-88, 1894.
33. Osler, W.: Dr. John Brown's spare hours. *Med News, 43*:273, 1883.
34. Osler, W.: *Elisha Bartlett, A Rhode Island Philosopher, with an appendix containing Dr. Bartlett's sketch of Hippocrates.* Providence, 1900.
35. Osler, W.: Silas Weir Mitchell, M.D., L.L.D. *Brit Med J, 1*:120-121, 1914.
36. _____ John Locke as a physician. *Lancet, 2*:1115-1123, 1900.
37. Cushing, H.: *Life,* vol. 1, pp. 221, 225.
38. Bay, J. C.: Conrad Gesner (1516-1565), the father of bibliography; an appreciation. *Papers Bibliographical Soc Amer, 10*:53-86, 1916.
39. Osler, W.: *Bibliotheca,* p. *xi,* No. 623.
40. Welch, W.H.: Foreword. In Abbott: *Bull Med 1*:641-642, 1913.
41. Osler, W.: John S. Billings, M.D. *Brit Med J, 1*:641-642, 1913.
42. _____ Address, in Memorial meeting in honor of the late Dr. John Shaw Billings. *Bull New York Public Library, 17*:516-518, 1913.
43. Cushing, H.: *Life,* vol. 1, p. 502; vol. 2, p. 249.
44. Osler, W.: Joseph Frank Payne, M.D., F.R.C.P. *Brit Med J, 2*:1751, 1910.
45. Osler, W.: An account of certain organisms occurring in the liquor sanguinis. *Proc Roy Soc, 22*:391-398, 1873-74.
46. _____ Foreword. In Vallery-Radot, R.: *The Life of Pasteur,* London, Constable & Co., pp. *ix-xx,* 1911.
47. _____ William Beaumont; a pioneer American physiologist. *JAMA, 39*:1223-1231, 1902.
48. Cushing, H.: *Life,* vol. 1, pp. 178-179, 590.
49. Bensley, E. H.: Alexis St. Martin. *J Mich Med Soc, 58*:738-741, 765, 1959.
50. Osler, W.: The leaven of science. In *Aequanimitas,* pp. 87-88, 1904; 3rd ed. pp. 82-84, 1932.
51. _____ Dr. William H. Welch. *American Magazine, 70*:456-457, 459, 1910.
52. _____Bates, D. G., and Bensley, E. H.: The inner history of the Johns Hopkins Hospital.

Johns Hopkins Med J, 125:191-192, 1969.

53. _____ Influence of Louis on American medicine. *Bull Hopkins Hosp,* 8:161-167, 1897.

54. _____ Impressions of Paris. *JAMA, 52*: 702, 1909.

55. _____ Alfred Stillé. *Univ Penn Med Bull,* 15:127, 1902.

56. Stillé, A., and Maisch, J. M.: *The National Dispensatory; Containing the Natural History, Chemistry, Pharmacy, Actions and Uses of Medicines . . .,* 2nd ed. Philadelphia, Henry C. Lea, 1879.

57. Osler, W.: Alfred Stillé, p. 132.

58. Osler, W.: An Alabama student. *Bull Hopkins Hosp, 7*:6-11, 1896.

59. Osler, W.: *Bibliotheca,* Nos. 4268, 4269.

60. Cushing, H.: *Life,* vol. 1, pp. 221-222, 409; vol. 2, p. 561.

61. Flexner, A.: *Daniel Coit Gilman: Creator of the American Type of University.* New York, Harcourt, Brace & Co., 1946.

62. Cushing, H.: *Life,* vol. 1, pp. 645-646.

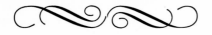

Essay VII

William Osler: The Egerton Yorrick Davis Alias

WILLIAM B. BEAN, M.D.

THE PENUMBRA CAST by William Osler's extraordinarily complex and challenging personality, with its characteristic lights and shades, has led his followers to concentrate on the light portion. Osler's assumption of an alias, though mentioned here and there, has not been confronted systematically. Since it is a characteristic of man's nature to be full of paradoxes, even great men may have important but unorthodox features of character and personality which need attention. It is my purpose to tackle Osler's imp of the perverse. An erratic sprite made him a perennial practical joker, provided a vehicle for his unquenchable ribaldry, and supplied many a nagging and not completely answered question in our efforts to evaluate the whole man.

Perhaps those who believe in omens might have read an important sign in the timing of William Osler's birth in Bond Head, Toronto, Canada. The date was the 12th of July, 1849. From the very time of

his birth, William Osler was singular in his manner of doing things. And it began with the selection of his name. His parents had intended to honor one of the patrons of the upper Canada clergy society and name their newborn son Walter Farquhar Osler. But little Willie, always ready and able, upset their plans by arranging to be born on the 12th of July. The choice was eminently shrewd since the Osler's region of Canada was distended with lusty Ulster Irishmen. Every year, on the 12th of July, these local Orangemen marched in formal procession waving orange and blue banners, riding white horses if they could, and making a gorgeous din. When they heard of the birth of a son to the Featherstone Oslers, the procession, in full panoply, marched on the Anglican parsonage. Thus, on that particular 12th of July when his father, beaming from the veranda proudly, held up the newborn babe for display, a cry went up in unison "William, William." The name stuck.

It is not surprising that Willie's older brothers and sisters assumed that there must be something special about him. Willie no doubt agreed, since each time his birthday came around a huge company repeated the pilgrimage, procession, and pageantry.

Willie was full of the small boy's mischief, though whether his juvenile transgression often went beyond what would have been accepted as tolerable in growing boys we do not know for lack of data from any controlled study.

But before the family left Bond Head, there were harbingers of the future. Indeed, Osler's medical career began in a very unorthodox way with a surgical operation. When he was five years old, at a large Sunday school picnic, Willie's family gave him the chore of chopping up kindling wood for the fire. Chattie, his then seven-year-old sister, kept teasing him by putting her finger on the chopping block. The five-year-old operator, after many and ample warnings, told her he would count three. If she did not remove her finger, he would chop it off. She didn't. He did. The exasperation was just too great. Only the tip came away, but it left her with an interesting scar by way of memento. Willie seems to have escaped any significant punishment since his weeping sister pled his case effectively by assuming the blame.

As the youthful favorite, he well deserved the nickname "Benjamin" which his mother gave him, though with his dark eyes he might equally well have been called "Little-Burnt-Holes-in-the-Blanket," which his father called him for a time.

The next year, when Willie was six, the family moved from the wilderness of Bond Head, where they had been for twenty years, to Dundas "Mountain," near Hamilton. The day the family was preparing to clamor aboard the train and go bag and baggage, the trip was postponed when Willie caught a severe cold. Possibly it was whooping cough. So the trip was delayed; mercifully, it turned out, since the train they were scheduled to take crashed through the rickety old bridge over the Desjardins Canal. More than a hundred passengers were killed in a memorable and

frightful calamity. This whole branch of the Osler family might have been wiped out.

In Dundas, Willie was forever getting into scrapes, but generally getting out as well. At the age of fifteen he was expelled from the Dundas grammar school, either because he and his fellow conspirators unfastened all the desks and hid them in an attic which he had reached through a trap door from the top of a stepladder, a feat showing considerable athletic prowess, or because one morning bright and early he locked a gaggle of geese in the classroom with the expected public health pollution and noise hazard. The uncertainty is not about his responsibility for both deeds. This was strong and clear, but rather it is, which was the final blow? Willie was joyful when he was given the sack. It didn't seem to bother his father particularly because, as he reasoned, after all the school was controlled by Methodists. Osler's mother, who was to live to reach her one hundredth year, seemed to have been much more worried about her son's occasional failure to write a thank-you note after a visit than she was over his high-spirited shenanigans and disciplinary problems in school.

He departed, then, for the Barrie grammar school. Here he managed to escape disaster in spite of his practical joking and almost scandalous clowning. But Osler as a prankster came of age in the original Trinity College School in Weston. One of the boarding pupils in school fell ill. The matron thought he was feigning illness. She used the rather unorthodox form of punishment or treatment and emptied a chamber pot over the unhappy lad's head. This immediately made her a special target in an open hunting season with Willie Osler leading the pack. This misguided old soul they locked in a room which was then nailed tightly shut. The chimney and the window had been sealed in advance. Then, a cross between chemical warfare and fumigation was contrived by piping into the room the smoke from an evil burning mixture of chemicals, leather, feathers, rubber, and spices, or whatever they could find.

It was apparently almost too effective. The lady was fetched out just short of suffocation, frothing at the mouth and crying for revenge. The generally staid Toronto *Globe* headlined "Pupils Turned Outlaws." The boys were captured by the local constabulary, docketed for battery and assault, and put in jail. William's older brother, Featherston, who not only had removed the "Jr." appendix from his name, but the terminal "e" as well, a rising young lawyer, defended the boys capably. He got them out of jail after they had spent a couple of nights, with a fine of one dollar each plus costs. The family probably thought it was hilarious, though the matron no doubt carried bitter memories still muttering imprecations.

At this stage of his career Osler had demonstrated an infinite capacity for taking pains and an imaginative skill, perhaps genius, for practical joking which often took the form of subclinical warfare and an almost exophthalmic mania for mischief. Rather surprisingly at this stage of Osler's life he got a sharp change in direction from two scholarly biologists, Johnson and Bovell, who mingled medicine and the ministry in varying sequences, degrees, and proportions. Willie had been designated as the family's contribution to the Church of England. Fortunately, his course swerved sharply. His deeply religious mentors, Bovell and Johnson, introduced him to the wonders of the microscope and the lure of biology. Thus the Church's loss became Medicine's great gain.

It would appear that the most learned psychiatrists and psychologists are as confused as anyone else in trying to explain what makes certain persons practical jokers. Young boys often torment their associates and other animals. When such behavior continues into adult life, it resembles the eternal adolescence of Peter Pan, shorn of innocence. Retribution for some deep hurt, escape from the secret sorrow of hidden tragedy, or simply perennial boyishness—which, if any, explain this morbid strain in Osler?

Osler might be considered a natural patron Satan for practical jokers whose imp of the perverse rides them with incorrigible gusto. Probably most people not afflicted with precocious senility at one time or another have felt vivacious joy in bawdy songs, ribald verse, and dubious limericks. In Cushing's memorable and moving *Life of Osler,* one senses his desire to tidy up, and perhaps Lady Osler's pruning or behind the curtains presence made the Osler of the Cushing biography seem almost a plastic saint. In some parts, at any rate, the resultant, in the horrid jargon of the day, is Cushingoid, or perhaps better Cushingesque.

But Osler was still inspired by his perverse sprite. Once upon a time, back in the Montreal days, there appeared Egerton Yorrick Davis, late Assistant Surgeon, United States Army, stationed on the Indian Reservation opposite Montreal. When Willie Osler was the young secretary of the dignified medical society of Montreal, he got a little tired of the local windjammers and their exaggeration of personal experiences. He put on the program a paper entitled "Some Peculiar Observations in Obstetrics Among the Caughnawaga Indians." Egerton Yorrick Davis was scheduled to present the paper but at the appointed meeting he did not show up. Before the restless company decided to leave, a messenger rode up on horseback and apologized breathlessly for the unavoidable absence of Dr. Davis. He was attending the squaw of the Indian chief who was in labor.

The doctors, not wishing to be completely disappointed, requested that Osler read the paper. He did. Many anomalous and scarcely ever heard of incidents were duly related. When the paper was finished, the secretary, Dr. Osler, sat back into his seat, and, after the perennial custom of secretaries, buried himself in paper work as he prepared to spend hours on minutes.

After the brief but dignified silence that followed the applause, some pompous person took the floor, thanked the secretary, and spouted extravagant nonsense, perhaps even manufactured on the spot. The local Münchausens indeed rather dimmed the luster of Dr. E. Y. Davis' contributions. The essayist was promptly elected a member, in absentia, and the society directed that the paper be sent to the *Medical News* of Philadelphia for publication.

In 1896, when Osler was forty-six years old, he attended the annual meeting of the Pediatric Society of Montreal, where he read a paper on the classification of tics, or habit movements. He blew in, unannounced, at the dinner one of his old friends was having for a Boston pediatrician and his wife. He pulled up a chair by the matron and asked what she had seen in Montreal and whether she had paid a visit to Caughnawaga. She had not. She seemed devoid of a sense of humor and he continued to describe the great new suburb across the river, built with the benefactions of a retired American army surgeon, E. Y. Davis, with beautiful parks, schools, theaters, paved streets, museums, and an especially fine hospital for children. He finished by

describing the sad end of Davis—drowned in the rapids—"drunk, they say." The unsuspecting couple spent much fruitless time searching for the mythical suburb. After they learned the sad truth, it is reported that they did not list William Osler among their special friends.

Sometimes Osler's outlandish antics described things which, though stranger than fiction, were true. Here is the famous story of the baby on the tracks which first appeared in the "Notes and Comments" section of the *Canada Medical and Surgical Journal, 16*:376-377, 1887-8.

Dr. Parvin's paper[1] on injuries to the foetus reminds me of an interesting experience which I had in the North-West in 1886, which is worth placing on record. Mr. Fred Brydges had kindly met our party at the Portage to take us over the Manitoba and North-Western Road, and he mentioned that two days before, a woman, while in the water-closet on the train, had given birth to a child, which had dropped to the track and had been found alive some time later. I was so incredulous that he ordered the conductor to stop the train at the station to which the woman had been taken that I might see her and corroborate the story. I found mother and child in the care of the station-master's wife, and obtained the following history: She was aged about twenty-eight, well developed, of medium size, and had two previous labors, which were not difficult. She had expected her confinement in a week or ten days, and had got on the train to go to see her husband who was working "down the track." Having a slight diarrhoea she went to the water-closet, and while on the seat labor came on and the child dropped from her. Hearing a noise and groaning, the conductor forced open the door and found the woman on the floor in an exhausted condition, with just strength enough to tell him that the baby was somewhere on the track, and to ask him to stop the train, which was running at the rate of about twenty miles an hour. The baby was found alive on the side of the track a mile or more away and, with the mother, was left at the station where I saw her. She lost a great deal of blood, and the placenta was not delivered for some hours. I saw no reason to doubt the truthfulness of the woman's story, and the baby presented its own evidences in the form of a large bruise on the side of the head, another on the shoulder, and a third on the right knee. It had probably fallen between the ties on the sand, and clear of the rail, which I found, on examination of the position of the hole in the closet, was quite possible. William Osler.

He recanted somewhat, for subsequently, on page 734,[2] he had the following to say:

The highly improbable obstetric tale which I told in the January number has been too much for the credulity of many of your contemporaries, and to their criticisms I meekly submit, knowing well that in obstetrics and gynecology I cannot lose a reputation for veracity; but I am glad to see that Mr. Brydges has come to my rescue and that much fuller details of this truly remarkable case have been published in one of the Manitoba papers and have been copied into a recent number of the New York *Medical Journal*. With the doctor who delivered the placenta and the conductor who found the child on the track I now leave the skeptics. William Osler.

But the real follow-up on this comes from the detective work done by C. B. Farrar as he reported in the *Canadian Medical Association Journal,* March 28, 1964, volume 90, beginning on page 781. There was such an event. The baby born in this unorthodox way later became known as Railroad Winnie. It was known she was born on a train, but exactly how, her parents tried to keep secret. Winnie had developed some brain injury at the time. As a schoolgirl she was a little lame. One leg was shorter than the other. She had an ophthalmos on one side. But she married and had a large family. Thus, the truth was stranger than fiction.

Further authenticity comes from George Blumer's report that one time when he was on the staff at Johns Hopkins he wandered into the main library and wished to make a note of something he had read. There was a large table in the center of the room and in its drawer he discovered a large unsealed manila envelope. This he opened and found a series of affidavits signed by the conductor and brakeman of a Canadian railway train relating to the birth of a baby. These had been collected by Osler and they tell the story of a young woman far advanced in pregnancy who had boarded the train. She had felt the pangs of labor coming on and a desire to move her bowels and so had gone to the toilet. In the trains of those days the toilet was simply an open metal tube, a kind of throne, crowned with a toilet seat. The young woman seated thereon had given birth to a child who fell through the hole along another and stranger birth canal to the track below. The distracted mother attracted the attention of the train crew, the train was stopped, and the baby was rescued unharmed, probably with nothing more than a few cinders imbedded in its buttocks since it had obviously not landed on its head. In recent years this has stirred up more than one flurry in Earle Scarlett's Zebulun Column in the *Archives of Internal Medicine*.

Such events as stuffing objects into the pockets of a clergyman leaning over the umbrella rack at the Athenaeum Club in London, or snatching a nurse's purse on a streetcar and paying everybody's fare only to return it the next day with a note of apology were, strangely, important elements of his nature and continued throughout his life.

A harmless variation of the practical joke was the deadpan tale of outrageous improbability. I quote from some notes my father made after one of the Saturday night meetings at the Osler house. Osler had doubted something in the medical history of a man who said that he had had jaundice at the age of fourteen and commented, "When I was six months old, the son of a Church of England missionary in the wilds of Canada, I was being fed in the pasture along with the other calves; while standing in front of the bucket full of milk, a big blazed-face bull calf came up and butted me over backward into the bucket of milk. I can see that calf as distinctly as I can see you now."

Dr. Joseph Pratt recounted the following anecdote:

Once I was present at a luncheon at the University Club in New York which Dr. Osler gave during a meeting of the American Association of Pathologists and Bacteriologists. The other guests were Dr. Councilman, Dr. J. G. Adami of McGill University, and Dr. William MacCallum of Johns Hopkins. It was MacCallum who started Dr. Osler off by asking the name of this delicious fish we are eating. "It is scrod," said Dr. Osler. "Scrod!" said Dr. MacCallum, "I never heard of it." (Dr. Osler speaking), "You know what a capon is; scrod is codfish that has received the same treatment. The production of scrod has become a thriving industry along the New England coast, as Councilman knows." Dr. Osler then went on to describe in detail. "The cod come up inlets from the sea in great numbers in the spring and are diverted into narrow, shallow troughs, from which they are removed by the nimble hands of trained workers, who quickly and skillfully castrate them. They are then placed in large vats of artificial pools of salt water. There, after a month or so, their flesh acquires a new and improved flavor. They are then shipped to market." MacCallum showed by his expression that he was deeply interested and thanked Dr. Osler for giving him this information. "It is most remarkable," he said, "and all new to me." None of the others made any comment; so MacCallum had no reason to doubt that this was a real addition to his store of knowledge.[3]

Once when Osler sent Hewitson, a McGill graduate who was on his staff at Johns Hopkins, to look something up in the library of the Philadelphia College of Physicians he told him as he left Baltimore, "Do drop in on my old friends Philip Syng Physick and Shippen and give them my love." Hewitson obviously knew nothing about these long dead historic figures and spent the better part of the day trying to run them down in Philadelphia, and only on returning to Baltimore did the reason for the failure become apparent.

Osler was a friend and an admirer of the well-known pediatrician Abraham Jacobi whom he dubbed "the lion head of the tribe of Juda." When Jacobi was seventy years old, in 1900, there was a commemorative dinner to celebrate the occasion of his birthday. Jacobi knew he would be called on to make some kind of speech and perhaps was a little nervous about this occasion. He had prepared a speech and had tucked it into the pocket of his coattails. As they were going upstairs to dinner, Osler, immediately following Jacobi, saw the end of the manuscript protruding from Jacobi's pocket and abstracted it as unobtrusively as a professional pickpocket. When Jacobi sat down to dinner he reached for the paper which was gone and his leonine head and massive brow became bedewed with cold sweat. Some minutes later and well before Jacobi had any occasion to speak Osler had a way to hand the manuscript to Jacobi with the explanation that it had been picked up on the stairs by one of the guests.

The furor of the "Fixed Period" address occurred under circumstances many of you know and led to a full-scale newspaper vendetta against Osler. A "practical" joke played some time before might have been bothering the memory of reporters, though the Baltimore press was notably restrained in reaction to the "Fixed Period" address.

Early in October 1904, Abraham Jacobi again was visiting the Oslers in Baltimore to give an address. Osler usually escaped reporters; but finally one of them managed to elude the delaying tactics of his Negro servant, Morris. He confronted Osler in his study, asking him for background material for an article about the distinguished visiting pediatrician from New York City. Jacobi was a small, hunchbacked man of leonine appearance, obviously Jewish. According to what I was told, Osler handed the reporter a photograph of John L. Sullivan, eminent practitioner of the pugilistic art, elbows bent and fists forward, in the ancient pose of the boxer. Other versions have it that Jacobi was described as a brilliant high jumper and pole vaulter, a star performer for the New York Athletic Club. The story and, for all I know, the pictures got into the newspapers. It is not recorded whether this scoop ended the professional career of the reporter, but it did create a stir.

So the "Delilah of the press" was ready for vengeance. Osler had been an outspoken critic of the often sensational and scientifically naïve lay press as it dealt with medical and scientific matters. Even today medicine has a cacophony of confused trumpet blowers among the many accurate and excellent writers. In any event, Osler was stalked by those looking for an opportunity to get even.

The Fixed Period is the name of a Trollope novel almost totally overlooked by scholars. It was published in 1882. Osler had read it years before he used the title "The Fixed Period" for his own farewell address to his students, colleagues, and friends when he left Baltimore to become Regius Professor of Physic at Oxford on Washington's birthday, February 22, 1905.

"The Fixed Period" was the year of grace given to colonists in a mythical country, to live on the bounty of the government and medicare from the age sixty-seven to sixty-eight. Then they were to commit suicide and be cremated. The substance of my comments this morning deals with this novel of Trollope which is somewhat more suggestive of Jules Verne or H. G. Wells, than the Warden, Barchester Towers, Phineas Finn and the other gentle reminders of the English rural scene of a hundred years ago.

Osler had the firm conviction that the great germinal work of the world had been done and could be done only by the young. He recognized that some creativity and especially the flowering of wisdom might occur in older people. But he insisted that "The teacher's life should have three periods, study until twenty-five, investigation until forty, profession until sixty, at which age I would have him retired on a double allowance. Whether Anthony Trollope's suggestion of a college and chloroform should be carried out or not, I have come to be a little dubious as my own time is getting short."

Now let us consider the book. Probably Osler first read Trollope's novel *The Fixed Period* when it was coming out in Blackwood's Magazine in the winter of 1881-1882, which was his last year in Montreal. Perhaps he read it in the two-volume English edition of 1882, or maybe in the Tauchnitz edition published in Leipzig.

During the Trollope revival after World War II, I met several Trollope scholars, none of whom had ever heard of *The Fixed Period*. In fact, it took me a good many years to lay my hands on a copy. I find some of Trollope's endless canters over the English countryside of a hundred years ago a little soporific but *The Fixed Period* is spiced with the mood of Jules Verne. Basically it is a study of how one's attitudes change with aging. We all recall how decades ago, someone much younger than we are now, seemed fearfully old. Our benchmark travels along with the calendar of our own years. Age and youth we reckon from the shifting parallax of our own personal chronology. One decade's old man becomes an older man's youth.

Trollope's story concerns Britannula, an imaginary island about the size of Jamaica, plopped down in the Pacific near where New Zealand is. It is settled by young rebels from England who judged most of the world's harm to be done by the elderly and the old. Among the many innovations of their new Utopia was a method for the elimination of old folk. The time of the story is roughly 1984, or about a hundred years after Trollope wrote it. *The Fixed Period* was approaching for the two main protagonists who as young men had founded a society for the prevention of the aged. Neverbend, the governor, and his friend approached "deposition." By laws they had enacted, the "College" of the colony was required to receive each citizen when he became sixty-seven years old. This was not Osler's mistaken recollection of sixty, and not sixty-three, the grand climacteric of the Romans, the 3 x 7 x 3. "Voluntary" suicide was not by chloroform but by the traditional Roman method of Seneca—immersing one's self in a warm bath, opening a vein and bleeding to death. This was the graduating ceremony at the end of the year of retirement-and-retreat at government expense and medicare. The spacious grounds of the college contained the very latest model of crematorium, a necessary adjunct to the Commencement Exercises. The college was called Necropolis. We would have called it Memory Gardens or Linger Longer Lodge.

As the story begins, the approaching need for the crematory is tested in a dry run where the bodies of huge pigs were used. By a fluke or faulty flue the cremation was heralded far and wide by an aroma which Bo-bo of Lamb's famous tale would have recognized at once. We should recall that in 1880 when Trollope wrote, the revival, or should I say resurrection, of cremation was looked upon by the intellectually hermaphroditic and emotionally overripe with as much enthusiastically misplaced queasyness as a few fur-wearing and meat-eating folk today look upon humane animal experiments.

The Britannulans had many innovations, including national cricket matches, with new rules and bigger and better teams. The ball was bowled by a mechanical steam bowler like the machines today's postulants in tennis or baseball may use for practice. Mountain climbers had mechanical arms to help them scale precipitous heights safely and rapidly. Steam tricycles had electric lights so they could be used at night. Something like instantaneous teletype recorded speeches anywhere in the world as they were delivered. How melancholy. Private talks danced across oceans or between shore and ship, all long before telegraph or wireless, telephone or television. The special surprise was Trollope's prophecy of a weapon like the atomic bomb. Indeed, Britannula was brought to heel by a British warship in the harbor, with a secret weapon. One blast from it could wipe out the metropolitan capital, the republic and all inhabitants. The constitution was revoked and the folly of youth trying to expunge old age was corrected.

Osler made this wry comment as the dust from the unexpected explosion began to settle.

It is an interesting experience to wake in the morning and find oneself "infamous"—the country ringing with criticism and the mails bringing reams of abuse. This is what happened to me on the twenty-third of Feburary. On the twenty-second I gave the University address and made it a sort of valedictory. I had always had the idea—and talked about it very much—that after forty no very great work was done. From Montaigne I think I got it. Then Anthony Trollope's novel, *The Fixed Period,* and a contemplation of the burdens, mistakes and calamities of old age had made me pick upon sixty as the age when a man should get out of harness. In my address I dwelt upon these two points, and in a humorous way spoke of the advantage it would be to universities if at the sixtieth year professors were made to retire into a college—as in "The Fixed Period"—for a year, at the end of which they would be quietly chloroformed, this being Trollope's suggestion. There was a great laugh, and I expressed my own doubt of the advisability of the scheme as I was myself approaching sixty. The exact words may now be read in the printed address, "The fixed period." That evening at the dinner we joked about it, but no one seemed to have thought anything very extraordinary had been said. The next morning, however, when the papers came out, the New York *Journal,* the *Herald* and the *World,* and the local papers! Big headlines, "useless at forty," Professor Osler recommends all at sixty to be chloroformed," Lethal chamber for the aged." The fat was in the fire. Such a row! The truth is I had had a big advertisement in the comments made upon my Oxford appointment, and it was a slack season for news. Newspapers, letters, clippings, poured in and within forty-eight hours things began to look serious. No paper contained a correct statement of what I did say, so I sent it in two or three paragraphs to the New York *Sun.* Then I cut the matter off—so far as it was possible. I read nothing more about it and refused all interviews. But it was a deuce of a row and I was more sorry for my friends than I can tell. Mrs. Osler was very worried but I had made up my mind to take Plato's advice and creep under the wall of silence until the storm blew over. The newspapers worked it as good material regardless altogether of the occasion or the actual words. I do not believe anyone took the trouble to give exactly what I said. One or two tried to be decent, the New York *Sun* and the New York *Post,* and E. S. Martin wrote some capital paragraphs in *Harper's Weekly.* "To Oslerize," "Oslerized" became common expressions. The hubbub did a good deal of harm, and I was heartily sorry for the many old people who were hurt by the outcry. Good came to a few—in stirring up the slackers and bringing the young men to work. I was pestered to death with reporters and for many months I could not sign my name in a hotel register. I kept a stiff upper lip so as not to let the thing get on my nerves, but it was an anxious and distressing time.

Osler was not the first, nor the last, to experience "the martyrdom of fame."

I am sure Osler felt that he was addressing only friends and family. Whether someone leaked the story or whether a reporter had been smuggled in or crept in no one knows. But the day after he presented what he thought was a friendly, perhaps not too painful, farewell address the journals, white, yellow and any other color, having little else

to concern themselves with, blasted banner headlines all over the country, "Osler recommends chloroform at sixty." He thus quite inadvertently was made to appear the enemy of the old. In almost the literal sense of the saying "he was hoist by his own petard." He made one or two rebuttals to the most gruesome misrepresentations, but then decided to let the matter die down if not die out.

I do not know that anyone has made a full collection of the Pseudonymous Papers published by Egerton Yorrick Davis. Besides the miscellaneous unpublished manuscripts of Egerton Yorrick Davis, M.D., late US Army, Caughnawaga, PQ, in the Osler Library, there are the following from Maude Abbott.

"Professional notes among the Indian tribes about Gt. Slave Lake, N. W. T., by Egerton Y. Davis, M.D., late U. S. Army Surgeon." This *jeu d'esprit* of Osler's was properly suppressed after being set up in proof for the *Canada M. & S. J.,* 1883. The MS. is in the Osler Library. It is prefaced by later "biographical" data: "I never could understand about Egerton Y. Davis . . . One thing is certain, he was drowned in the Lachine rapids in 1884, and the body was never recovered . . ." (see Cushing, "Life", i, pp. 240-1). In other words, his disappearance coincided with Osler's departure from Montreal.

Vaginismus. (Correspondence, signed "Egerton Y. Davis, Caughnawaga, Quebec"), Med News, Phila., 1884, xlv, 673. Inspired by the editorial, *ibid.,* pp. 602-3, this is still seriously quoted as the Davis case! Though Osler wrote it, he was not responsible for its publication. It was vouched for by the editor of the *Canada M. & S. J.,* who sent it to the *Med News* in revenge for the trick Osler had played on him the previous year (see above).

Extra-uterine changed into intrauterine pregnancy by electricity.[4]

Peyronie's disease—Strabisme du pénis. (Correspondence, dated "Pittsburgh" and signed "J. W. W., Jr.") *Boston M. & S. J.,* 1903, cxlviii, 245. A genuine case of LaPeyronie's disease, whimsically reported by Osler over the initials of his friend J. Wm. White, of Philadelphia, who humorously proves its Baltimore origin in a letter,

Ibid., p. 485, which White signed with Davis' initials, misprinted "E. T. D., Jr."

Then there is a review of "Diseases of the Liver, Gall-Bladder, and Bile-Ducts. By H. D. Rolleston, M.A., M.D. (Cantab.), F.R.C.P., Physician to St. George's Hospital, London; Formerly Examiner in Medicine in the University of Durham; and Fellow of St. John's College, Cambridge, England. Fully illustrated. Philadelphia, New York, and London. W. B. Saunders & Co., 1905."

The Egerton Yorrick Davis alias dies hard and one sees often enough in contemporary journals Egerton Yorrick Davis spoofing somebody or other. I receive letters regularly from two friends who have had a life long interest in Osler which they may or may not sign Egerton Yorrick Davis or E. Y. D. as the mood seizes them. In *Natural History,* volume 56, 1947, there was interesting correspondence dealing with men being swallowed by whales in an outlandish letter from Boston in a series of letters telling of fascinating episodes of men alleged to have been swallowed by whales. In his charming current book, *The Year of the Whale,* Victor B. Sheffler reviews this correspondence. He dealt with the whole thing in a tongue-in-cheek or man-in-whale-mouth fashion. From time to time, friends of mine have accused me of using the E. Y. D. alias myself. I have never elevated myself to the pinnacle of plagiarizing Osler's alias nor have I sent anonymous letters, however much I might have been tempted to do both.

CONCLUSIONS

In describing the E. Y. D. aspect of our hero, and my most particular medical hero, William Osler, I come neither as muckraker nor iconoclast. We must never let the enshrining of heroes become an apotheosis

in which deification, ascribing superhuman qualities to a human being, takes him out of the simpler sphere of hero worship to the worship reserved for the divine. So, as I have done on a good many occasions in speaking of Osler, or writing of him, I wind up this potpourri by quoting two paragraphs from the earlier paper, dealing with part of the same subject.

I should like to conclude with a personal parenthesis. Isn't it curious how the printed word passes most of us by most of the time and many always. Every now and then it produces astonishing effects as unconsciously and as unobtrusively as the seed planted by a teacher. Osler's words to medical students about measuring nail growth started me twenty-five years ago on a study still in process of the growth of my own thumb nail. The nail still grows, albeit, more slowly. You have heard about this. Osler's casual sentence concerning Daniel Drake awakened an interest which has led me to collect a substantial number of Drake's books. Osler's comments about rare diseases started me down another garden path of singular and abiding interest. Osler's words on Dunglison and dictionaries— "After all there is no such literature as a dictionary," accounts for six lovely old dictionaries on my shelves. But the longest pilgrimage which at odd intervals took me into dozens of libraries and many more bookstores finally led me to a copy of Trollope's *Fixed Period* which you have heard about.

The conclusions of even a brief talk often fall between anticlimax and supererogation. To me Osler was no paper saint, but a very human person. His imp of the perverse sustained a streak of practical joking which made many people miserable and got him into a world of trouble. The main point of his life, though, was that he was able by hard work and self discipline to forge the powerful instrument of character which was and is a model for physicians all over the world. He made the realm of clinical medicine his own and so enriched his age. He recognized the essential continuity of life in biology, science and medicine and, thus, let history interpret for us the present in terms of the past. By doing so he helped us learn to use history and not to be ambushed by it. We who live in troubled times, which is to say with every age "today," owe fealty to a hero who was indeed a person with the human qualities we all have, but beyond this, he had purpose and dedication. By such simple attributes as work, drive, order and persistence, he burnished his talents into subtle but shining skills. Their reflection lights our way as we try to combine knowledge with care and wisdom with *caritas,* hoping, thus, to become better physicians and better men.

REFERENCES

1. Parvin: *Med News, li*:561, 578, 1887.
2. *Ibid.,* p. 734.
3. *Proc Inst Med Chic, 26*(No. 6):138, 1966.
4. *Med News, 48*:279, 1886.

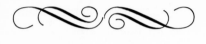

Essay VIII

Excerpt from "An Uncatalogued Paper Published by William Osler in 1902"; The First Presidential Address of the American Osler Society

WILLIAM B. BEAN, M.D.

In pursuing the Osler-Reed association, I chanced upon the forgotten Osler paper which was published next to Walter Reed's paper in a group of tributes to Dr. W. W. Johnston, a distinguished Washington clinician and teacher who was admired and loved equally by his patients and colleagues. Osler's paper is characteristic of his skills, his high ideals, his insistence on professional standards, and his generous admiration and praise.

DR. JOHNSTON AS A PHYSICIAN
by
WILLIAM OSLER, M.D., LL.D.
Baltimore, Maryland*

IN HIS CHARACTER as a physician a man has a threefold relation with the public, with the profession and with himself. Not one of us in all, only a few of us in some of these diverse relations, live up to our full capacity. In an exceptional degree our departed

*Washington Medical Annals, 1:158-161, 1902.

friend was faithful to this triple allegiance.

The public of today makes it increasingly difficult for the physician to walk in the old paths, and yet we cannot afford to abate one jot or tittle from the noble standards of the Hippocratic code, that most memorable of human documents. What a blessing it is to our fellow creatures to feel that they can go freely to the physician and unburden tales of weakness and of woe, which not even the confessional receives! And it is one of the chief glories of our profession that in every age we have held high this standard of honor, and have inspired and deserved this sacred trust. Dr. Johnston had in singular measure this gift of inspiring confidence. A firm but gentle manner, decision of voice and of character, unfailing kindness and a rare knowledge of the symptoms and treatment of diseases, combined to make him a practitioner of the very first rank. And this confidence he never abused. He neither pandered to the press, which is always too ready to tempt the prominent physician to tickle the itching ears of a gossip-loving generation with prurient or spicy details of cases; nor did he trade upon the credulity of his patients, but *caute caste et probe* dealt as an honest man with his suffering fellow creatures.

A physician's relations with his colleagues may be widespread and intimate, or they may be of the most restricted kind. There are doctors in large practices who, without the slightest sense of responsibility, live secluded from all professional inter-course. In the midst of an active profes-sional life it becomes increasingly difficult to keep up an interest in teaching, in medi-cal societies and in medical literature; but, as you will hear, in all these lines Dr. John-ston worked with energy and zeal. I may refer briefly to his literary and scientific work. Influenced strongly at secondhand through his father by the French school, and directly by J. Hughes Bennett, he very early learned the art of careful observation. The tribute he paid to his old teacher, Bennett, one of his last papers, showed clearly that he was his model, and a better [one] it would be hard to name. *The Trans-actions of the Association of American Physicians,* of which he was an original member, contains a series of important papers from his pen. He was particularly interested in the subject of fevers, and there were few men in the country who had a wider and more varied experience with typhoid fever. On dysentery and its treat-ment, he had written at intervals for many years, and the last and most comprehensive work on the subject is to be found from his pen in a recently issued volume of *Wood's Reference Handbook.* On the whole ques-tion of intestinal diseases he was an ac-knowledged authority, and the articles which he contributed to *Pepper's System of Medicine* are among the most complete and scholarly in that encyclopedia.

To the very last he had the strong feeling that a man was a debtor to his profession, and amid the distractions of an unusually exacting winter he was busy working at the subject of bronchiectasis. In the persistency with which he thus kept in touch with the productive section of our guild, he left an example which many of us could follow with advantage. I wish there was a general clearing house to which such men as Dr. Johnston could report, say every second or third year, a sort of central committee which might skim the cream off the experi-ence of such men and present it to the profession. The difficulty is that the young write too much, the mature too little. There is too much green fruit sent to market, and the fruit of too many of the fine trees is never plucked at all.

In no relationship is the physician more often derelict than in his duty to himself. I do not refer so much to the sins of care-lessness of health and improvidence of time which so easily beset us, nor to that self-sacrificing devotion to patients which has broken many a strong man in the full strength of his maturity. Dr. Johnston in these matters was one of the chief of sin-ners, as he never spared himself, but in one respect he earned the encomium "well done, good and faithful servant." There are un-pleasant features about the parable of the talents, but it has an application in the life of our friend. With his environment and heredity he could have wrapped his talent in a napkin and left it quietly in the same case with his parchment, but instead he had a keen sense of responsibility, and sought the usury to be had only by study and by the laborious days and nights of the student. What gave him personally a special value was the confidence we, as a profession, felt that his experience was a genuine product, not the bastard variety which twenty-five years of practice may give to any man with an imperturbable countenance and a glib tongue. The public still follows the old saying about Drs. Maybe and Mustbe: "Remember, the young doctor may be experienced, but the old doctor must be. You take no chance with Dr. Maybe when

Dr. Mustbe is in reach." Nothing can be more fallacious than the current belief that years of practice bring experience. All depends upon the type of growth, whether endogenous or exogenous. The mere accretion of facts, the daily routine of cases, is not and does not bring experience. It is the man's attitude toward these facts. The men in whom we have confidence, to whom we turn in difficulties, are those who have correlated the events of the daily round, and who have digested and assimilated mentally the raw products of experience. To do this seems (indeed, to some men it is), an easy matter, even amid a routine of a most exacting kind; others only do it as a bounden duty. To bring out of the treasures of a full-stored mind things new and old to bear upon the individual case, to know when to act with vigor and promptness, to recognize when to hold the hand, to distinguish between the victory of nature and the triumph of art—these were qualities of mind which increased in our friend with the growing years.

So much dies with him that the death of a man of Dr. Johnston's experience and influence is, for a time at least, an irretrievable calamity in a community. In scores of families there are aching hearts for the good physician and warm friend who had been so faithful in the hour of need, whose place may be taken, but can never be filled. Students mourn a teacher whose example was an inspiration, and who made them feel the dignity and honor of the calling of their choice. The Profession of the District of Columbia lament the loss of a man in whose position they took a pride, whose best efforts were always at their disposal and upon whom they had learned to lean as a trusted counselor. And, speaking for a larger body, I may express the deep regret of his confreres of the Association of American Physicians, and of his colleagues, the teachers of medicine throughout the land, at the loss of so distinguished an ornament of our beloved profession.

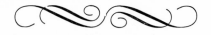

Essay IX

Osler and War

ALFRED R. HENDERSON, M.D.

ONE COMMON AND PROMINENT trait among the eminent of history has been the possession of heroes in their minds and hearts whom they worshiped and emulated. Sir William Osler had his heroes, and he wrung them dry of their wisdom, learned from them, looked up to them, borrowed from them, and with their aid became, as he quoted from John Milton, "the complete man to perform all the offices, private and public, of peace and war."[1]

Few have been so affected by the lives of others, those by whose example he set the stance and gait of his own thought and action. Portraits of Linacre, Harvey and Sydenham hung together in prominent view above his fireplace. But as much as he revered these men, there was another above them all, possibly too close to his own time to be as often quoted, Louis Pasteur. Osler called him "the most perfect man who has ever entered the kingdom of science."[2] In common with Pasteur, who had directed the students of the University of Edinburgh to "worship great men," Osler had an equal reverence for the illustrious dead.

Osler embarked early in life with Sir Thomas Browne as a traveling companion and with his wise words: "In the virtuous voyage of thy life ye shall not go about like an ark, without the use of rudder, mast or sail: expect rough seas." And Sir Thomas'

"Quiet them our commotions" became Osler's oft quoted "consume your own smoke."[3]

In these times of intensive application of man to war and other diverse forms of strife, it is more than just a matter of candid interest to literally ransack the lives and counsel of those we cherish as "heroes." What was Osler's attitude on war, its causes and attendant problems? How did this ideal exemplar of both classic and moral humanism, with a deep reverence for life, think and react to war? He loathed it! He called war a malady, "a periodic attack of acute mania, a bad one, too,"[4] and ". . . a dirty and bloody business, worthy of the Oxydracians, who by the means of Levin-bolts and thunder, more horrible, more frightful, more diabolical, maiming, breaking, tearing, and slaying more folk, confounded men's senses and threw down more walls than would a hundred thunderbolts."[5]

Bred the missionary's son, with a biblically oriented childhood and youth, and raised in a day when many hours a week were devoted to the Scriptures and every fiction had a moral ending, he credibly stated, "Our young minds are trained to regard warfare as one of the prerogatives of Jehovah, the Lord of Hosts, who 'teachest my hands to war and my fingers to fight'."[4]

And what does a man think and do who has been raised to extol and even worship as acts and intercessions from on high the battles and battlers of the Old Testament? Can all wars be wrong when the Lord purposefully set up the adversaries of Rezin against him and joined his enemies together for battle? (Isaiah 9:2) And did not the Lord direct the military operations of David against the Philistines, and smite them from Geba to Gazer? (I Samuel 5:22-25) And how does this sound to those who would confine their belief to a weak-kneed, namby-pamby God: "And I will bring distress upon men, that they shall walk like blind men, and their blood shall be poured out as dust and their flesh as the dung"? (Zephaniah 1:17) And this: "And I will set my face against you, and ye shall be slain before your enemies; they that hate you shall reign over you, and ye shall flee when none pursueth you"? (Lev. 26:17) Osler may have been, as he said, "nurtured on the Old Testament," but Osler, the man, was well seasoned with the New Testament as well. Early in life he learned to leaven his religion with the yeast of humanism in its classic meaning and temper it with the "lives and lips" of early teachers. The character that came out of all this need not be dwelled upon here, for an Oslerian is an Oslerian because he is already familiar with the heart and head of the man. Osler's views on war, as with every other thing, are best viewed by the example of his life.

There are three distinct greater qualities in the character of Osler. I do not refer to those readily noticeable attributes pointed out by Penfield, "the least sentimental, the most helpful and the most lovable teacher of medicine."[6] Nor do I mean the "sunny disposition and dolphin-like delights" written about by Viets,[7] or the 261 qualities of personality catalogued by Davison.[8] I speak in a deeper sense of the quality of imperturbability or equanimity, the quality of detachment and the quality of humanism, in the Christian sense. With these three major qualities uppermost in mind let us

witness how the thorough and proper disciplining of a young life carried the older man through those portentous, soul- and body-trying years of World War I, the "war to end all wars."

One of the Osler family recently wrote, "Equanimity he learned from his mother, who had been more concerned with his failure to write a 'thank you' note than she was over his various troubles with school authorities."[9] Osler took the meaning of the word *aequanimitas* from the quality of the life of Antoninus Pius, as portrayed by Marcus Aurelius:

Have a care you have not too much of a Cesar in you . . . be candid, virtuous, sincere and modestly grave . . . justice and piety have their share in your character; let your temper be remarkable for mildness and affection . . . imitate him (Antoninus) in this . . . *equality,* sweetness and piety of his temper, his contempt of fame . . . dismiss nothing until you look through it and move it on all sides . . . be not at all apt to be frightened, not too suspicious, firm in friendship . . . pleased with a better expedient than your own. To conclude, he was a religious prince, but without superstition. Pray, imitate these good qualities of his, that you may have the satisfaction of them at your last breath as he had.[10]

Was this not also Osler?

How many other scholars through the centuries have waded knee-deep through the *Meditations* without stamping the life of Pius with a single word upon the lives of succeeding generations? Of the three varieties of the famed—creators, transmuters and transmitters—Osler said, "Man owed his world dominion to the transmitters,"[11] and to this Cushing added, "the inspirers and animaters."[12] To this class we relegate Osler for placing this word *equanimity* in our working vocabulary.

To what reaches can one practice equanimity? Is feeble, calamitous and miserable man limited in his capacity to control his temperament when all of Selye's stress mechanisms are rocketing his adaptive physiology toward the point of disintegration? The hysterical and shocked, the "effort hearts" and "psychical decerebrations" that were returned from across the Channel gave sufficient proof that there exists all grades of stamina and resistance and persistence in men in this regard.

As with most wars, the onslaught was swift and gave full evidence of methodical German planning; within a few days in August 1914, Luxemburg, parts of Belgium, France and Russia were occupied. Within a week, Germany, Austria and Italy, and France, Russia and Great Britain had declared war on each other. The suddenness of being struck was quickly followed by inevitable confusion in an unprepared England and, permeated by fears, rumor and unfounded opinion quickly displaced fact.

I know of nothing that Osler had said or written which revealed any pre-war anxiety or any warnings that war was imminent. He noticeably kept out of politics and rarely mentioned anything concerning world affairs, in spite of numerous and ample warnings about Germany's increasing military strength.

The twentieth century had opened with great promise and enthusiasm for progress in every aspect of human endeavor. During the latter nineteenth century, " . . . science emptied upon him (man) from the horn of Amalthea blessings which cannot be enumerated, blessings which have made the century forever memorable, and which have followed each other with a rapidity so bewildering that we know not what next to expect."[13] Osler was optimistically caught up in the age of growth everywhere. "These are glorious days for the race. Nothing has been seen like it on this old earth since the destroying angel stayed his hand on the threshing floor of Aranuah the Jebusite."[14] He stated this in 1909, amid the warnings

of a farsighted unheeded few who were accused of seeing Germans beneath every bed, and while a myopic foreign relations group in the Cabinet was demanding large-scale reductions in military spending. Trafalgar Square and similar places began to witness anti-war, anti-mobilization, peace-at-any-price demonstrations by students, labor and liberal groups, which were continued even after the war began. Andrew Carnegie's peace speech at Liverpool and Lord Haldane's enlightening discourse before the University Extension Course at Oxford, explaining the ethnological and other mutual differences between Germany and England and how a better understanding of the German mind might diminish the differences of opinion, had, of course, no influence upon Germany's long-planned aggression. Lord Haldane went to Berlin in early 1912 to engage in friendly and confidential communications with those responsible for Germany's policies, and his chatter was accompanied by the dredging clatter at the Kiel Canal which was being enlarged to accommodate the new German battleships.

Osler, reflecting later on those pre-war days, stated, "And yet in what a fool's paradise many of us have been living, flaunting in the face of history our wish for peace—seeking it, ensuing it, with the war-drums throbbing in our ears."[4] "We shut our eyes to the beginnings of evil," wrote Amiel, "because they are so small, and in this weakness lies the germ of our misfortunes."[15]

It seems now almost incredible that a man so vitally concerned with the peace and concord and unity of man, and who would have been the first to have detected a public health hazard and to have acted on it, seemed so oblivious to the signs of impending war. There are, obviously, perils in detaching oneself so wholly from the political scene.

And so it was that while the Third Hague Peace Conference was being planned, Germany became the only nation prepared and geared for war. Henry Van Dyke, then United States Minister to the Netherlands, described the era:

It was like watching a stage curtain which rises very slowly a little way and then stops. Through the crack one could see feet moving about and hear rumbling noises; evidently a drama was in preparation. Then, after a long wait, the curtain rose swiftly. The tragedy was revealed . . . and caught France dozing along the Luxemburg border with hardly enough guns there for a big rabbit shoot.[16]

In early June of 1914, Van Dyke, while fishing a bordering trout stream, had noticed and reported the day-long movement southward of German troop trains from Köln to Trier.[16] When the holocaust came, Osler was vacationing at the Strathconer's island retreat and planning a trip to the United States.

The initial response in Great Britain was to "hate the Hun," "damn the Kaiser." Such responses reflected an intense exasperation as much as pure hate, heightened by the embarrassed state of unpreparedness. But peripatetic Osler was not caught up in this mass hostility. His first recorded statement was made in a letter to Mrs. Brewster, friend of Baltimore days: "What a mess," he wrote, "it all seems very unnecessary, but the nations are still in the nursery stage." Then, prophetically, his United States trip postponed, "I am so disappointed not to see you all. But it is a small matter in comparison with the tragedies that are inevitable in the families of friends."[12] Immediately, he became concerned about his many friends in Germany, a concern he kept throughout the war. "He was a little naive, possibly in regard to some of the consequences of the war," wrote Cushing, "and could not believe that it would affect either

the friendship or the humanitarian attitude of individuals on whichever side they might be."[12] While there was never any doubt about the origins of the war and the guilt of the German Emperor and his military forces, Osler kept blameless the many good German people, and particularly his professional friends, who were as much caught up in the "horrible mess" as he was.

Within a month of the outset of war, a syndicated letter appeared in Allied newspapers addressed to "The Civilized World," and obviously put there by the German Propaganda Office.[17] The open letter was signed by ninety-three leading scientists of Germany, many of them close friends of Osler. The purpose of the letter was to help convince the world that Germany was not responsible for the war and to ". . . protest to the civilized world against the lies and calumnies with which our enemies are endeavoring to stain the honor of Germany in the hard struggle for existence . . . in a struggle which has been forced upon her."[17]

A letter of response soon appeared, composed by Lord James Bryce, former Ambassador to the United States and later Chairman of the Atrocities Committee, and signed by 116 of England's leading scientists, including Osler.[17] In the "Reply to the German Professors by British Scientists," it was regretted that so respected a group, for the most part, could have added their names to such a document. "We can hardly believe that it expresses the spontaneous and considered opinion of those who live under a Government which, we believe, does not allow them to know the truth," it added.

There is ample evidence that suspicion that the German professors had little or nothing to do with this letter was correct. Paul Ehrlich of Frankfort, one of the "signers," had declared at the war's beginning: "But this war is pure madness! No good can come of it."[18] From the beginning of the war, his Serum Institute had been taken over and controlled by the Government.

"I am very sad about all my good German friends. I wonder where the truth lies? Bottom of an artesian well these times," wrote Osler early in the war.[12] In his address, "The War and Typhoid Fever," given in November 1914, Osler compared the necessary fight against war diseases by the great army of sanitation with the " . . . needless slaughter of the brave young fellows, Allies and foes alike."[19] He simply did not know who to hate, and he continued to write letters of condolence even to Germany, as to Frau Professor Ewald in Berlin on learning of her husband's death.[20]

Osler had always had a high regard for German science, and one cannot but wonder if, after 1914, his own remarks of an earlier time, 1894, returned to him in a disquieting remembrance. He had been speaking of the need for good laboratory men,

. . . men with ideas, men who have drunk deep of the Astral wine, and whose energies are not sapped in the treadmill of the classroom . . . Germany must be our model in this respect. She is great because she has a large group of men pursuing pure science with unflagging industry, with self-denying zeal, and with high ideals. No secondary motives sway their minds, no cry reaches them in the recesses of their laboratories, "Of what practical utility is your work?", but unhampered by social or theological prejudices, they have been enabled to cherish the truth which has never been deceived.[20]

When the German wounded began to arrive at the Oxford Hospital, he remarked, "The German wounded came in last week . . . fine looking fellows, all of them."[12]

Much later in the war, during the great German drive of the spring of 1918, when for a time things looked black for the Allies, Lady Osler wrote, "The conditions in France have depressed him dreadfully—we talk freely of visits from the Müllers and

Ewalds should the Huns reach England."[12]

Osler just could not include his old friends on the continent with the "Gott Strife England" class. "What a cruel shame the rulers have made outlaws of such good people as we know—at least in the profession," he wrote to Henry Hurd. "I wish they would hang a few of the newspaper editors . . . there will be an awful Gulf between this country and Germany for the next two generations. Their hate is nothing to the loathing expressed here on all sides . . . unfortunately, there seems to be no question about the Belgian horrors."[12]

Osler knew firsthand about the Belgian horrors, for after the occupation and sacking of Louvain, with total destruction of the famed University Library, twenty-one Belgian refugee professors and their families had found shelter at Oxford in the care of the Oslers. Thus, another project came to occupy the Oslers, that of finding clothing, food and support, and even work, for these destitute refugees. Countless letters went out to friends in America and Canada appealing for both cash and materials for their care.

Osler was made an Honorary Colonel in the Oxford Regiment, but did not make a good soldier in the military sense. He ordered the wrong kind of uniform, but did not change it and throughout the war he dressed, when absolutely necessary, in the uniform of a major. He did not like to wear his uniform, but found it a very necessary thing to do when making visits to the military hospitals.[12] It would seem that Osler upheld the dictum of Machiavelli that "Scholars are never good soldiers, which a certain Goth well perceived for when his countrymen came into Greece, and would have burned all their books, he cried out against it, by all means they should not do it; leave them that plague, which in time

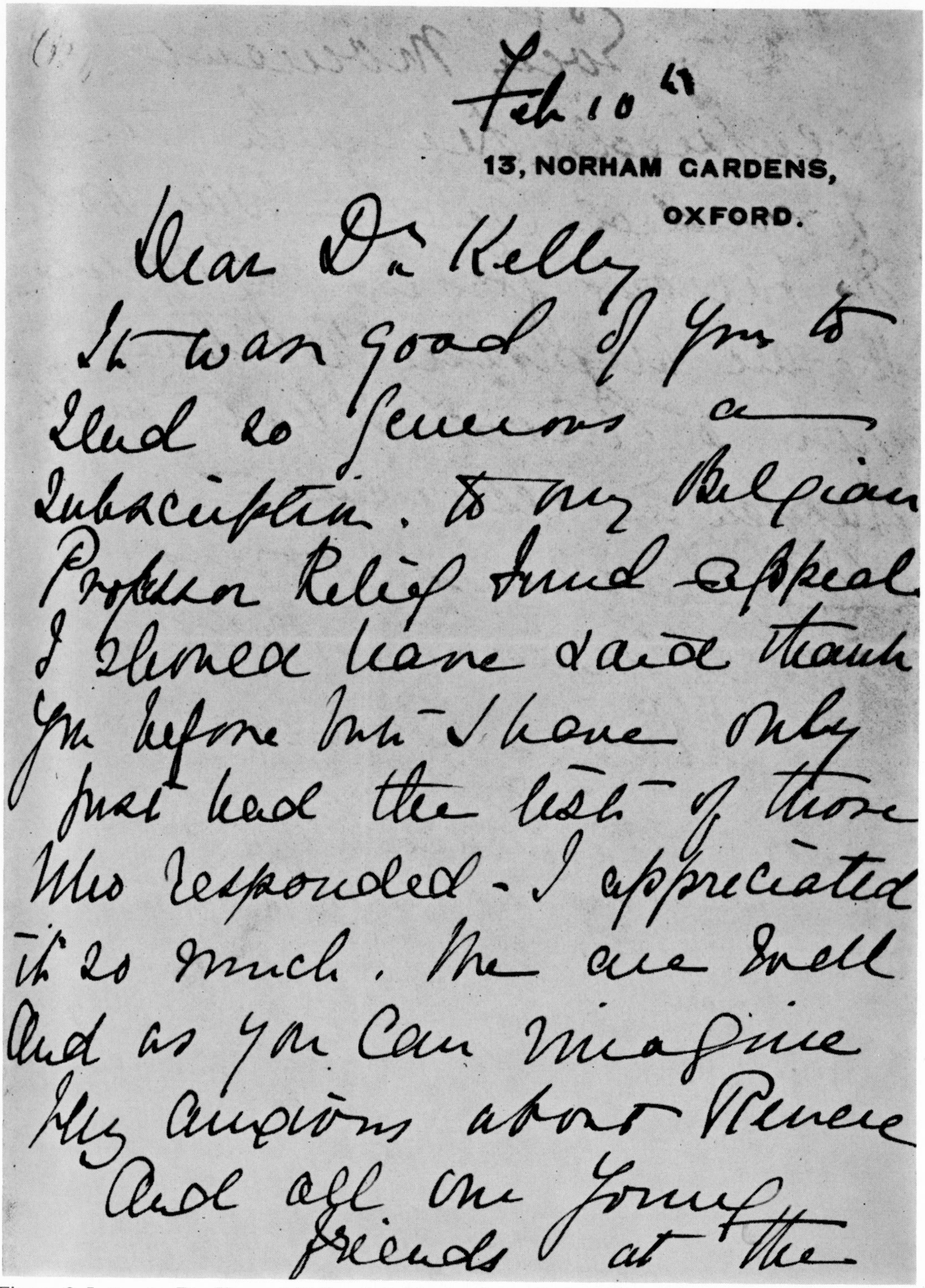

Feb 10"

13, NORHAM GARDENS,
OXFORD.

Dear Dr Kelly
It was good of you to
lend so generous a
subscription. to my Belgian
Professor Relief fund appeal
I should have said thank
you before but I have only
just had the list of those
who responded. I appreciated
it so much. We are well
And as you can imagine
very anxious about Revere
And all our young
friends at the

Figure 2. Letter to Dr. Howard Kelly of Baltimore from Lady Osler, February 12, 1917: "It was good of you to send so generous a subscription to my Belgian Professor Relief fund appeal . . , we are well and as you can imagine very anxious about Revere and all our young friends

fronts - Every moment is
occupied here with the
wounded and war work
in various forms. Of course
we are anxiously waiting
now to know what will
happen in America -
My husband joins
in affectionate messages -
Always Sincerely
Grace R. Osler.

at the front. Every moment is occupied here with the wounded and war work in various
forms. Of course we are anxiously waiting now to know what will happen in America . . ."

will consume all their vigor and martial spirits."[21]

While others could talk of nothing other than the war, Osler would not permit conversation of this kind and seldom read the newspapers. "Open Arms," his Oxford home, was something like a railway terminal at times with friends and friends of friends partaking of the warm hospitality to be found there. Frequently, members of the Canadian Expeditionary Forces, American voluntary medical units, and other military personnel were guests in the home, with fresh news and views of what was going on in the war. Osler would have none of it and would divert their attention to other things, especially his library and medical history.

But no one worked harder at war than did Osler, and none worked harder to get others to work. He put the "master word" *work* to use as never before. With this magic word all things did seem to become possible with him, but at the cost of much of his life's energies, when other men of comparable age did more resting and cogitating than working. Later, with his own son in the midst of Flanders' fighting, his words of the past took on real meaning, ". . . the absorption in the duty of the hour is in itself the best guarantee of ultimate success in avoiding the disastrous effects of worry."[22]

As his voluntary war efforts occupied more and more of his time and strength, there was less time for private consultations and less income. Where the pages of his account book formerly were filled with appointments for consultations, he kept pencilled notes of his wartime activities and thoughts.

Even with the daily news of new weapons and horrors of war, brought to him most realistically by his own contact with the maimed in the hospitals, he remained apart from the antipathy of the mass of the people, the master of his emotions. During chapel services at Oxford commemorating the University losses at war, he considered the mockery of such memorial services and confessed, "I could not help thinking of the nice German women singing this afternoon, 'Ein fester Burg ist unser Gott,' as I used to hear them in the cathedral in Berlin."[12] Shortly after this, in characteristic detached manner, he wrote to L. L. Mackall in America, who was preparing to return to the continent to resume his studies, "If you have the chance, give my hearty greeting to the Ewalds in Berlin and to the Müllers in Munich."[12] Had not his mentor, Sir Thomas Browne, said, "While we look with fear or hatred upon the teeth of the viper, we may behold his eye with love"?

In an apparent calmness, Osler reflected upon the menace about him. In an address given at Leeds Medical School, October 1, 1915, he said,

The explanation is that we are still in the childhood of civilization. Some millions of years divide the Tertiary period, when man broke away from the great ape stock, and the dawn of our modern era . . . In time our civilization is but a thin fringe like the layer of living polyps on the coral reef, capping the dead generations on which it rests. The lust of war is still in the blood, we cannot help it.[4]

Revealing his reluctant acceptance of war, he continued, "There was and there is as yet, no final appeal but to the ordeal of battle . . . Let us remember, too, that war is a human development, unknown to other animals."

The well qualified student of human nature knew, indeed, what he had to accept. The apathy of the Baltimore city officials against reforms in public sanitation, the dead-ends encountered in establishing tuberculosis reforms in America, England, Ireland and Wales, and combatting of resistance to needed reforms in medical education and certification in both America and Great Britain, were all comparatively weightless by comparison with what the war years demanded and received of him.

Osler had found the key to a full understanding of the etiology of war in the wisdom of his ancient heroes and mentors. In thinking of Osler, one cannot help but recall the poem dedicated to him by S. Weir Mitchell, "Books and the Man":

> Show me his friends and I the man shall know,
> This wiser turn a larger wisdom lends;
> Show me the books he loves
> And I shall know the man,
> Far better than through mortal friends.[23]

What did his Master, Plato, say about this malady of mankind? "It seems to me," stated Plato, "to have thought the world foolish in NOT understanding that war is always going on among all men and cities. For what men in general term peace is only a name; in reality, every city is in a natural state of war with every other . . . no one can be a sound legislator who orders peace for the sake of war, and not war for the sake of peace."[24]

In considering the war's beginnings, one must agree with the master historian of war, Thucydides, who commented that, "No one ever plunged headlong into war from ignorance of what will follow—nor yet when they expect to gratify their ambitious views are they ever deterred by fear."[25]

Man's state of immaturity dominated Osler's thought in speaking of conflict. In his "Old Humanities and the New Sciences" address, Osler stated to a young generation, newly overseasoned with science, ". . . in the mystic shadow of the *Golden Bough*, and swayed by the savage emotions of our ancestors, we stand aghast at the revelation of the depth and ferocity of primal nature."[5] And to dispel any ideas his young audience might have that any revelations in the de-

veloping sciences will ever really do much for man, he continued,

The leaven of science gives to man habits of mental accuracy, modes of thought which enlarge the mental vision and strengthen . . . the sinews of understanding. But is there nothing further? Apart from science, we are apt to forget those things beyond her domain . . . those irresistible forces which alone sway the hearts of man. With reason, science never parts company, but with feeling, emotion, passion, what has she to do? They are not of her. Science may have chained lightning, but who has chained the wayward spirit of man? . . . no leaven, earthly or divine, has worked any permanent change in him. "At all ages, the reason of the world has been at the mercy of brute force and never can have more than that so long as man is human. The individual intellect, the aggregate intelligence of nations and races have alike perished in the struggle of mankind. To relive again, indeed, but as surely to be again put to the edge of the sword."

A vast amount has been written concerning human aggression since the Great War to "end all wars." Unknowledgeable but opinionated, flame-red scribblings from pastel-pink brains, the sociologists and psychologists only serve to expand their own bibliographies and confuse the issues on war. They would do themselves immeasurable good by taking their start from Osler's notion of man in his nursery stage and to thoroughly digest the most scholarly work of all time on war, *De Jure Belli ac Pacis*, written by Hugo Grotius, a contemporary of William Harvey, in that intellectual season of seasons, the early part of the seventeenth century.[26] What a refreshing academic breeze it would be to see a simple, unemotional and unentangled explanation of how wars are caused by an idiot, or group of megalomaniacs with too much (but never enough) power, committing the act of coveting something they have no right to! The sophisticated theories concerning the differences between groups of people, cultural, socio-economic, racial, religious, genealogical or any other antipathy never explain the cause for war.

Osler, fully understanding the primitive motives of the enemy-aggressor, also knew that to resist this evil and to render him beaten and punished was not primitive or evil but the only mature, manly and credible response. Thucydides has given the correct answer to aggression:

> It is, indeed, the part of the wise, so long as they are not injured, to be lovers of peace. But it is the part of the brave, if they are injured, to give up the enjoyments of peace, that they may enter upon war, and as soon as they are successful, to be ready to sheathe their swords. Thus, they ought never to allow themselves to be too much elated by military success, nor yet be so fond of peace, to submit to insult.[27]

Let us not for a moment interpret Osler's quality of equanimity as being related in any way to pacifism. No man with Plato as mentor, and a well-worn Bible at his elbow, no activist such as Osler could be a pacifist, or as Cushing added, ". . . or a fool."[12] "There is a shrewd remark in the *Republic*," wrote Osler, "that the most gifted minds, when they are ill-learned, become pre-eminently bad."[28]

The mind of the pacifist and the so-called conscientious objector were 'pre-eminently bad minds' to Osler, who cast himself wholly into the war, like Sir Thomas Browne, "not with the armour of Achilles, but with the armature of St. Paul."

As he reflected upon war, Osler wrote, "Crile was right in his conclusions about man." George Crile had written in his book, *A Mechanistic View of War and Peace,* "Although this war was precipitated by certain nations, its fundamental cause is to be found in no one nation alone; for every nation, race and tribe has waged war . . . war is a normal state of man."[29] Crile believed that the noncombatant, the pacifist, is more emotional than the combatant.

Osler's unique ability to disjoin, or de-

tach, himself from his immediate environment was a lasting and useful trait throughout his life. You will recall him as a small schoolboy, reading his lessons while squabbling friends were romping all about him, with his fingers stuffed in his ears to keep out the noise. Everyone familiar with his life knows well how he could turn abruptly from a distressed situation and plunge himself into his library and books or turn about and play with small children, becoming even as one of them. Perhaps someone can explain the cybernetic phenomena involved in this kind of mind. It may be wholly true, from a more gross point of view, that the studies carried out on his brain in 1928 revealed little of unique anatomical interest. However, the day is approaching when perhaps more modern ultramicroscopic and chemical analysis may show more.[30]

In 1915, during his visit to the battlefront, standing amid the squalid spectacle of what had been farms and villages, surrounded by the noise and all that makes up the battlefront setting, he paused and, looking heavenward at the planes being shot at, simply stated, "What a scene!"[12]

When the zeppelins dropped bombs on England, with the resultant panic and death that occurred, he calmly wrote, "Things are going well for the country. The Zeppelin raids are a great stimulus, and so far the damage is below the Lusitania level."[12] The zeppelin raids, in fact, were a big adjunct to recruiting.

He worked hard to avoid thinking. He was a consultant to every military hospital within reach and regularly attended the Radcliffe Infirmary, daily except on Monday and Friday. Every Monday he paid an official visit to the wounded at the Duchess of Connaught's Hospital on the Astor estate at Cliveden, a forty mile automobile trip. He was a frequent visitor, to both patients and staffs, at Canadian and American camps and hospitals. From the very beginning of the war, he lectured to these encampments on war diseases and the need for innoculations against typhoid, which was not mandatory for the military at that time. On Fridays he visited Mt. Vernon where, due for the most part to his own efforts, an Army Heart Hospital had been constructed. Then back by noon for Oxford University Press board meetings. The Shorncliffe Army Hospital and the Colchester Heart Hospital were also frequently visited by him.

In addition to all this, he wrote editorials to newspapers, bolstering the hopes and dispelling the fears of a mass of people close to war. It was a common occurrence for his articles and editorials to appear in American medical journals. These writings served to inform the profession abroad, not yet caught up in the conflict, concerning the medical problems of war. His letters reflected his ever-dominating optimism, invariably ending with a brief sentence, "All goes well here and looking brighter. The spirit is at high pitch and we are all in it and all goes well with us here." "How splendid Canada is doing!"

Osler saw war as a vast opportunity for an education that could not be gotten under any other circumstances and he utilized the war for this purpose to its fullest extent. When weary from duties far in excess of what almost anyone else was doing on the home front, he would not complain. He

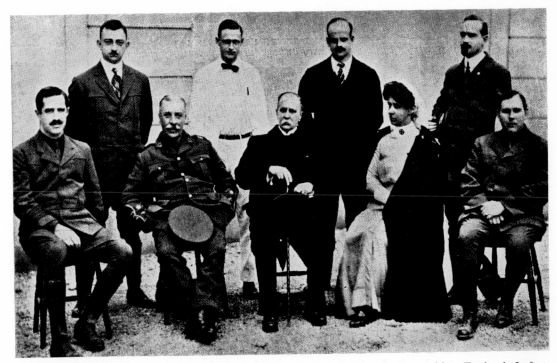

Figure 3. Staff of the American Woman's War Hospital, Paignton, S. Devonshire, England. Left to right, standing: Dr. J. L. Stowers, Dr. W. T. Fitzsimmons,* Mr. Hosmer, Dr. Edgar L. Gilcreest; seated: Dr. R. W. Hinds, Lt. Col. Gunning, Sir William Osler, Head Matron, Dr. William Crunnley. (Courtesy of the Smithsonian Institution photographic collection). *First American killed in the A.E.F. The Fitzsimmons General Hospital, Denver, Col. is named for him.

would only remark something about how hard war was on the younger fellows. ". . . it's a terrible strain on the young men," he commented to Henry Viets.[31]

To attempt to enumerate Osler's wartime work here would leave room for nothing else. As the war years dragged on, the battlelines almost permanently set and the cost of a few kilometers of dirt taking thousands of lives, he grew a little less patient. An added strain was President Wilson's chronic indecision and America's status of "armed neutrality." Indecision and neutrality were untenable to Osler's thinking. To remain neutral, or to be a pacifist, in the face of the war's atrocious history betrayed a severely crippled manhood. Osler felt the need for America to be in the war from its earliest weeks. On September 15, 1914, his wife had written, ". . . he is sending letters and books to President Wilson and all the prominent men about Germany's lying attitude."[12] America's neutrality created a dual role for Osler, rallying American consciences abroad and allaying English bitterness at home. Among those whose martial spirit he helped to arouse in America was an old Philadelphia friend, J. William White. Dr. White, Clinical Professor of Surgery at the University of Pennsylvania, carried on his own little war among the neutrals. He raised over five thousand dollars for Lady Osler's Belgian refugee fund, collected both money and supplies for the American Ambulance Hospital in Paris, and wrote and published a "Primer of the War for Americans."[32] Osler took it upon himself to distribute the "Primer" among influential persons in civil and government life. ". . . 'tis a hard thing to stir a democracy," he wrote to J. J. Walsh.[12]

Stirring a democracy that is well informed and topped with a manly leadership, that separates politics from matters of life and death, is not difficult. But when the Chairman of the Foreign Relations Committee, William J. Stone, who was voted into office by a large German population in St. Louis, can compel the Secretary of State, William J. Bryan, to issue an official letter denying any Administration unfriendliness to Germany and partiality to Great Britain, the confused democracy is, indeed, difficult to stir.[12] "If we only had a President who was a man," wrote H. C. Wood, from Philadelphia, "Roosevelt would have settled this thing months ago!"[12]

As the seemingly unprogressing war dragged on there were occasional glimpses of the wearing down of a little of Osler's equanimity. In a letter to J. William White he went so far as to insert, "D. the K.!" And to George Dock he wrote the only fringe-profanity I have ever encountered from his pen: "I am afraid we are in for a long business. Germany is far from defeat and the U. S. will have to give the knockout blow . . . Tell the damned pessimists to shut up. I am ashamed to meet them— there are a few here who growl that not enough is done."[12]

He must have felt his own temperament sorely tested. "Not a pacifist, but a 'last-ditcher!' . . . Two years changed me into an ordinary barbarian."[5] By this time there was more than the ordinary circumstances of war to test him. His son Revere was at the front in Flanders and no fewer than fifty of the Canadian branch of the family were in uniform, eighteen at the front. Of these derivatives of Featherstone Lake Osler and Ellen Free Pickton, four were wounded, one gassed, one a prisoner, one shell-shocked, and two were killed. The Oslers were so well represented in the services that an editorial appeared in a Toronto paper entitled "The Osler Volunteers."[12] The Oslers, disposed to peace, echoed Kipling's lines when the need came:

For all we have and are,
   For all our children's fate,
Stand up and take the war,
   The Hun is at the gate![34]

The long awaited Allied offensive, which broke the two and a half year stalemate plight of both sides in the Flanders salient and which had worn the combatants down to almost insupportable low levels of morale, got underway on July 31, 1917. Enlish, Scottish, Irish and Welsh troops, aided on their left flank by French remnants of the 1st and 51st Divisions, entered the German lines at all points of attack. In the sector where Edward Revere Osler's Battery A, 59th Brigade, operated, the Steenbeck River was crossed and held between St. Julien and Landmark. The artillery followed close on the heels of the infantry, where they regrouped and awaited the command to move further eastward through German occupied land when the weather cleared. The best laid plans of mice and men, the greatest battle of the war thus far, the Third Battle of Ypres, was halted by mud. "The weather joined the enemy" wrote Buchman, and the battleground became the "spongy salient."[35] Although the misery of ground-fast troops, under these circumstances, cannot be pictured in words, General Douglas Haig put it succinctly, "The low-lying clouds, the claying soil, torn by shells and sodden by rain, turned to a succession of vast muddy pools. The valleys of the choked and overflowing streams were speedily transformed into long stretches of bog, impassable except by a few well defined tracks, which became marks for the enemy's artillery."[36] Stopped short, as they were, Revere and his battery were looked down upon by the German Batteries eastward on the Passchendael Ridge.

Prophetically, on August 19 Lady Osler

had written to Harvey Cushing, on learning that he and Revere were located near the same front, ". . . how badly you would feel if you should see him brought in wounded; but what a mercy it would be for him."[12] In his journal, August 30, 1917, Cushing wrote, "Rather used up, I was preparing to turn in at 10 last night, when came this shocking message: 'Sir William Osler's son seriously wounded at 47 C.C.S. Can Major Cushing come immediately?'"[37] The battery had taken a direct hit from over the Passchendael Ridge. There were other American doctors serving as volunteers at nearby base hospitals and receiving stations who knew Osler, and were soon found at Revere's side. Crile, Eisenbrey, Darrach and Brewer were there, but talent, transfusion and surgery failed to save Revere. In the early morning of August 31, Revere was buried in a soggy Flanders field, wrapped in a weather-worn Union Jack. "A strange scene," wrote Cushing in his journal, "the great-great-grandson of Paul Revere under a British flag, and awaiting him a group of some six or eight American Army medical officers—saddened with the thoughts of his father."[37]

When the message reached Osler he was busy in his library, working on the new edition of his textbook. In his notebook he wrote: ". . . a sweeter laddie never lived, with a gentle and loving nature . . . and was devoted to all my old friends of the spirit—Plutarch, Montaigne, Browne, Fuller . . . Izaak Walton . . . we are heartbroken, but thankful to have the precious memory of his loving life . . ."[12]

His first response was to shield others, his wife, his friends. "Poor Grace! It hits her hard; but we are both going to be brave and take up what is left of life as though he were with us."[12]

That she and William might have at least

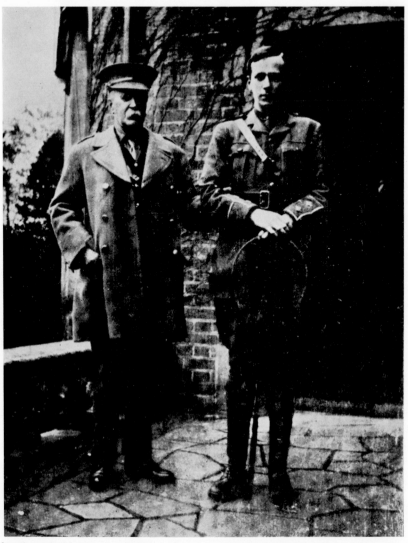

Figure 4. Colonel and Lieutenant Osler. (Courtesy of the Osler Library, McGill University).

one day alone at home, Lady Osler wired, cancelling his engagements. A visiting Swiss physician failed to receive the message, came to lunch and stayed until late afternoon. Only upon his return to the station did he learn from the chauffeur of Revere's death. Dr. Whitelocke told of meeting Osler that afternoon in the corridor of the Acland Home and of Osler calling out, "Hello, Whitelocke, how's my dear boy getting on?" Dr. Whitelocke was so taken aback that he did not realize that it was his own son, Hugh, whom Osler was asking about. When he told Osler that his son had come down with dysentery in the Middle East, Osler replied, "Be sure and let me know if I can do anything for him. You'll be glad to know that poor Revere fell into the hands of some American friends. Such a comfort. Do keep me posted about Hugh. Goodbye, old chap."[12] In wonderment, but with an aching heart, Dr. Whitelocke turned to watch him pass down the corridor, "not a trace of emotion—a lesson in manliness, restraint and breeding."

On the following day he made his rounds at Taplow, as usual, going through the wards in the same gay way. "But when he got to the house for luncheon," wrote Nancy Astor, "he sobbed like a child—it was so hard for us who loved him."[12] He did not, even now, show a personal animus toward the Germans, nor would he allow others to do so in his presence. He knew who the real enemy was, it was the innate primitiveness of man that permitted war to happen; his enemy was war.

By all outward appearances he was back to work as usual, "only with a sore heart." His books, the small children of his friends, and hard work occupied his mind during the day, but his nights were ghastly for a long while. How often his very own words, uttered early in the war before his own sorrow, must have returned to him, "Humanity has but three great enemies, fever, famine and war; of these by far the greatest, by far the most terrible, is fever."[38] Was it fever, after all?

John Tyndall once preached to his students, "The formation of right habits is essential to permanent security. They diminish your chance of falling when assailed, and they augment your chance of recovery when overthrown."[39] This meeting has been devoted to a life that exemplifies this counsel. What more perfect example can one find that illustrates the practical, down-to-earth, workable consequences of proper breeding? Add to this parent-imparted acquisitiveness to worthy heroes in early life, heroes to serve throughout life as ready counsel and a supporting scaffold against the storms that invariably blow. Osler understood the nature and the causes of war as lying within the fine ground structure of man, a remnant function of his still maturing species. Man's admirable developments in science and education had nothing to offer him in solving his behavioral enigmas, indeed, science has only served to make wars more devastating.

And for those who would replace faith and a soul with cold science, pause briefly and listen to these wise words of Omar Khayyám, penned some seven and a half centuries before us:

> Khayyám, who stitched the tents of science, has fallen in grief's furnace and been suddenly burned; the shears of fate have cut the tent ropes of his life, and the broker of hope has sold him for nothing.[40]

A war later, musing over ruined and impoverished Germany, Charles A. Lindbergh wrote:

> The Germans, too, had been an educated people, with western minds and hearts. Few nations had contributed more to our civilization in the past—in art, music, religion, philosophy, science . . . millions of Germans had devoted their lives to the discovery and development of scientific knowledge . . . they worshiped science. To it they had sacrificed the quality of life—yet they had

Figure 5. Letter to Dr. James Tyson, Philadelphia, from Osler, September 14, 1917: "You will have seen the sad news of Revere's death on the 30th. The Battery was moving position and heavily shelled and seven of them were hit. Revere was taken to the nearest casualty clearing station, where fortunately he fell into the hands of Darrach and Brewer of New York who operated. Severe wounds of the chest and abdomen. Harvey Cushing arrived in time to be with him at the end. He only lived 16 hours. It is a terrible loss to us but we shall try to face it bravely . . . I had expected this all winter as the Battery has been in all the heavy actions of late and the Major in command has been wounded four times." (From the Author's collection).

See Double Page Spread 〉〉〉〉→

14 IX 17

13, NORHAM GARDENS,
OXFORD.

re death of his son

Dear J. T.

You will
have seen the sad news
of Reveres death on the
30th. The Battery was
moving position & heavily
shelled & seven of them
were hit. Revere was
taken to the nearest Cas-
ually-clearing station,
where fortunately he fell
unto the hands of Darrach &
Brewer of New York. who
operated — severe wounds
of chest and abdomen

Harvey Cushing arrived in time "to be into him" at the end. He only lived 16 hours. It is a terrible loss to us but we shall try to face it bravely. He had developed into such a fine stalwart fellow & so full of interest in the brighter & better things of life. I had expected this all winter as the Battery has been in all the heavy actions of late & the Major in Command has been wounded four times. Revere kept wonderfully well & has done the work very cheerily. I hope you are keeping well. Love to you all

Yours ever,

Wm Osler

not gained the power to survive . . . Perhaps survival, in the last analysis, was fully as dependent on the quality of life as on the power of arms—dependent on a perpetual balance of spiritual and material forces.[41]

The key, then, lies in the quality of *man,* still a recessive trait for the most part.

Osler wrote,

The history of man is the story of a great martyrdom—plague, pestilence and famine, battle and murder, crimes unspeakable, tortures inconceivable, and the inhumanity of man to man has even outdone what appear to be atrocities in nature . . . There is no place for despondency or despair. As for the dour dyspeptics in mind and morals who sit idly croaking like ravens, let them come into the arena, let them wrestle for their flesh and blood against the principalities and powers represented by bad air and worse houses, by drink and disease, by needless pain, and by the loss annually to the state of thousands of valuable lives, let them fight for the day when a man's life shall be more precious than gold . . . an approach to the glorious day of which Shelley sings so gloriously:

Happiness,
     And science dawn though late upon the earth;
Peace cheers the mind, health renovates the frame;
     Disease and pleasure cease to mingle here,
Reason and passion cease to combat there.
     Whilst mind unfettered o'er the earth extends
Its all-subduing energies, and wields
     The sceptre of a vast domain there.[42]

And *there,* wars will be no more.

REFERENCES

1. Osler, W.: An address on the hospital unit in university work. *Lancet, 1*:211, 1911.
2. Vallery-Radot, R.: *The Life of Pasteur,* translated from the French by Mrs. R. D. Devonshire; with a Foreword by Sir William Osler. London, Constable & Co., vol. 1, p. *xvi,* 1911.
3. Browne, Sir Thomas: Christian morals. In Sayle, C. (Ed.): *The Works of Sir Thomas Browne,* Edinburgh, John Grant, vol. 3, 1912.
4. Osler, W.: *Science and War,* Oxford, The Clarendon Press, 1915.
5. Osler, W.: *The Old Humanities and the New Science,* Boston, Houghton & Mifflin Co., 1920.
6. Penfield, W.: Hero worship. *Arch Intern Med, 84*:105, 1949.
7. Viets, H. R.: Osler and the tongue-tied medical student. *N Engl Med, 260*:822, 1959.
8. Davison, W. C.: The basis of Sir William Osler's influence on medicine. *Ann Allergy, 27*:370, 1969.
9. Osler, W. E.: The Oslers of Ontario: *Chatelaine* (Ontario), *43*:44, 1970.
10. Marcus Aurelius: *Meditations,* Book VI, of Miller, Marion Mills (Ed.): *The Classics, Greek and Latin.* New York, Vincent Park & Co., vol. VII, p. 67, 1909.
11. Osler, W.: Creators, transmuters and transmitters. In Keynes, G. L. (Ed.): *Selected Writings of Sir William Osler.* London, Oxford University Press, 1951.
12. Cushing, H.: *The Life of Sir William Osler,* Oxford, The Clarendon Press, vol. 2, 1925.
13. Osler, W.: Medicine. In *The Progress of the Century.* New York, Harper Brothers, p. 173, 1901.
14. Osler, W.: *The Treatment of Disease,* London, Henry Frowde, Oxford University Press, p. 5, 1909.
15. Amiel, H. F.: *Amiel's Journal, The Journal Intimé* (translated with introduction and notes by Mrs. Humphrey Ward), London, MacMillan Co., vol. 2, p. 76, 1885.
16. Van Dyke, H.: Pro patria. In *The Works of Henry van Dyke,* New York, Charles Scribner & Sons, vol. 11, p. 311, 1921.
17. *The New York Times Current History of the European War,* New York, The New York Times Co., vol. 1.
18. Marquardt, M.: *Paul Ehrlich,* New York, Henry Schuman, p. 239, 1951.
19. Osler, W.: The war and typhoid fever. *Br Med J, 2*:909, 1914.
20. Osler, W.: The leaven of science. In *Aequanimitas with Other Addresses,* 3rd ed. Philadelphia, The Blakiston Co., p. 92, 1952.
21. Machiavelli, in Burton, R.: *Anatomy of Melancholy* (Dell, F. and Smith, P., Eds.), New York, Tudor Publishing Co., p. 259, 1941.
22. Osler, W.: The master word in medicine. In *Aequanimitas with Other Addresses,* 3rd ed. Philadelphia, The Blakiston Co., p. 364, 1952.

23. Mitchell, S.W.: Books and the man. In *Complete Poems of S. Weir Mitchell*. New York, The Century Co., pp. 418-422, 1914.

24. Plato: *Laws*. I:626.

25. Thucydides: *Calamities of War*. IV:59.

26. Grotius, H.: *The Rights of War and Peace* (Campbell, A. C. and Hill, D. J., Eds.), New York, M. Walter Dunne, 1907.

27. Thucydides: *The Peloponnesian War*. I:120.

28. Osler, W.: Physic and physicians as depicted in Plato. In *Aequanimitas*. Philadelphia, p. 53, 1952.

29. Crile, G. W.: *A Mechanistic View of War and Peace*. New York, Macmillan Co., pp. 4, 39, 1917.

30. Donaldson, H. H. and Canava, M. M.: The study of the brains of three scholars: Granville Stanley Hall, Sir William Osler, Edward Sylvester Morse. *J Comp Neurol, 46*:1-95, 1928.

31. Viets, H. R.: A roving commission: The doctor calls on some of his friends. *Bull Hist Med, 22*:364-368, 1948.

32. Repplier, A.: *J. William White, A Biography*. Boston, Houghton & Mifflin Co., p. 229, 1919.

33. Bryan, W. J.: United States fair to all: Disclaimer of bias against Germany and Austria, (Washington, January 20, 1915). In *The New York Times Current History of the European War*. New York, The New York Times Publishing Co., vol. 2, pp. 1175-1183, 1917.

34. Kipling, R.: For all we are. In *The Writings in Prose and Verse of Rudyard Kipling*. New York, Charles Scribner's Sons, p. 18, 1920.

35. Buchman, J.: *A History of the Great War*. Boston, Houghton & Mifflin Co., n.d. vol. 3, p. 589.

36. Boriston, J. H. (Ed.): *Sir Douglas Haig's Dispatches, December 1915-April 1919*. London, J. M. Dent Sons, p. 116, 1919.

37. Cushing, H.: *From A Surgeon's Journal, 1915-1918*. Boston, Little, Brown & Co., p. 197, 1936.

38. Osler, W.: Bacilli and bullets. *Br Med J, 2*: 569, 1914.

39. Tyndall, J.: An address to students. In *Fragments of Science*. New York, D. Appleton & Co., chap. 5, 1871.

40. Omar Khayyám: *The Rubáiyát* (Edw. Fitzgerald translation), New York, Three Sirens Press, n.d., p. 16.

41. Lindbergh, C. A.: *Of Flight and Life*. New York, Charles Scribner's Sons, p. 18, 1948.

42. Osler, W.: *Man's Redemption of Man*. New York, Paul B. Hoeber, pp. 9, 60-63, 1915.

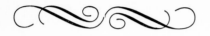

Essay X

Osler's Public Travel Letters: An Exercise In Humanism

CHARLES G. ROLAND, M.D.

BETWEEN 1874 AND 1915, a period almost spanning his professional career, William Osler wrote for publication at least twenty letters recounting his thoughts and experiences while abroad.[1-20] My purpose today is to present for you an impression of Osler as a humanist, principally by using Osler's own words from his public travel letters.

The letter from abroad was a common literary mode in the late nineteenth and early twentieth centuries. Leafing through the journals of the day, today's reader may begin to wonder if every medical visitor to a foreign land felt obliged to report back to his colleagues. But in those halcyon days without radio and televison I believe that the travel letter served a real role in communication.

Before going further I must indicate what I mean when I speak of Osler's humanism. First, I do not refer solely to the philosophical movement of humanism, the system which predominated in the period about 1400 to 1650 A.D. It is both unsafe and unrealistic to suppose that anyone, living

two and a half centuries after a philosophical system was at its height, can be considered an adherent of that system. That is, humanism today is not the humanism of Montaigne's time—scarcely a surprising observation. Nor is the humanism of 1970 identical to that of Osler's time; today, for example, we have a mundialized humanist movement with a central organization and an activist attitude which I suspect Osler would have difficulty accepting if he were with us now.

Perhaps the fundamental point is that Osler was not a philosopher in any deep sense of that word. Nor did he claim to be. We approach the flavor of his humanism, I believe, when we consider some of the other English words which share the same root. For Osler was *humane,* and believed in humaneness as a way of ordering one's life. And he concerned himself intensely with humanity in general and in particular. Nor was he exceeded by any physician of his time in his interest and support of the *humanities.*

Bergan Evans, in *The Natural History of Nonsense,* claims that any man who abandons or suspends the questioning spirit, even for one minute, has for that moment betrayed humanity. Osler never abandoned the questioning spirit. It is displayed in the first letters, written during a lengthy trip to Europe for postgraduate training; of course,

82

he should have had the spirit then, for he was young and eager. But he still had it when he wrote the last of these letters, when he was sixty-six years old. He describes his studies of rare functional nervous disorders, which he blames on "the extraordinary stress and strain of the trench fighting." Later I shall discuss in more detail Osler's views about war as they are displayed in these letters.

This audience needs little reminding of Osler's compassion and humanity. Yet I feel I must cite one anecdote from Cushing's *Life of Sir William Osler,* to provide an aura of this aspect of his character. Cushing mentions a time in 1875 when Osler dined with a young Englishman visiting Montreal on business.

One evening, observing that he appeared ill, Osler questioned him, and suspicious of the symptoms, got him to his rooms and to bed, where it was soon evident that he had malignant smallpox. The disease proved fatal after an illness of three days, and having learned the young man's name and address of his father in England, he wrote:

"My dear Sir, No doubt before this, the sorrowful intelligence of your son's death has reached you, and now, when the first shock has perhaps to a slight extent passed away, some further particulars of his last illness may be satisfactory. On the evening of Thursday 22nd, & on the following day, I discovered unmistakable evidence of the nature of his disease. On Saturday in consultation with Dr. Howard—the leading practitioner of our city, his removal to the smallpox Hospital was decided upon. I secured a private ward & took him there in the evening.

"Even at this date was seen the serious nature of the case, & I sent for Mr. Wood at his request. At 10 PM I found him with your son, & we left him tolerably comfortable for the night. He was easier on Sunday morning, but well aware of his dangerous state . . . After 11 o'clock he began to sink rapidly, & asked me not to leave him. He did not speak much, but turned round at intervals to see if I were still by him. About 12 o'clock I heard him muttering some prayers, but could not catch distinctly what they were . . . Shortly after this he turned round and held out his hand, which I took, & he said quite plainly, 'O thanks.' These were the last words the poor fellow spoke. From 12:30 he was unconscious, and at 1:25 AM passed away, without a groan or struggle. As the son of a clergyman & knowing well what it is to be a 'stranger in a strange land' I performed the last office of Christian friendship I could, & read the Commendatory Prayer at his departure.

"Such my dear sir, as briefly as I can give them are the facts relating to your son's death."

Thirty years almost to the day after this letter was written, the newly appointed Regius Professor of Medicine in Oxford chanced to meet at dinner a Lady S———, who, attracted by his name, said that she once had a young brother who had gone out to Montreal and had been cared for during a fatal illness by a doctor named Osler, who had sent a sympathetic letter that had been the greatest possible solace to her parents: that her mother, who was still living in the south of England, had always hoped she might see and talk with the man who had written it. Later, on his way to Cornwall, Osler paid a visit to this bereaved mother, taking with him a photograph of her boy's grave, which he had sent to Montreal to obtain.

This thoughtfulness and solicitude identify the best side of Osler. Yet I do not propose that a man is a humanist simply because he is kind—even though kindness is certainly an important element. Another hint of Osler's humanism is his contempt for chauvinism in science, an attitude he expressed positively by promoting internationalism in medicine throughout his life. Thus in one of his earliest letters, written from Berlin in November 1873, when he was twenty-four, Osler comments favorably on the fact that "at a Lecture the other day . . . representatives from Russia, England, Brazil, the United States and the Dominion sat peacefully next each other."[2]

Where chauvinism became virulent nationalism Osler did not hesitate from speaking out forcefully. Ten years after he wrote the preceding letter, he visited Berlin again; he found a repugnant situation, and wrote back to Canada critically:[5]

The modern *"hep, hep, hep"* shrieked in Berlin some years past has by no means died out, and, to judge from the tone of several of the papers devoted to the Jewish question, there are not wanting some who would gladly revert to the plan adopted on the Nile some thousands of years ago for solving the Malthusian problem of Semitic increase. Doubtless there were then, as now, noisy agitators . . . who clamored for the hard laws which ultimately prevailed, and for the task-masters whose example so many Gentile generations have willingly followed of demanding, where they safely could, bricks without straw of their Israelitish brethren. Should another Moses arise and preach a Semitic exodus from Germany, and should prevail, they would leave the land impoverished far more than was ancient Egypt by the loss of the "jewels of gold and jewels of silver" of which the people were "spoiled." To say nothing of the material wealth—enough to buy Palestine over and over again from the Turk— there is not a profession which would not suffer the serious loss of many of its most brilliant ornaments, and in none more so than in our own . . . The number is very great, and of those I know, their positions have been won by hard and honorable work; but I fear that, as I hear has already been the case, the present agitation will help to make the attainment of University professorships additionally difficult. One cannot but notice here, in any assembly of doctors, the strong Semitic element; at the local societies, and at the German Congress of Physicians, it was particularly noticeable, and the same holds good in any collection of students. All honor to them!

Yet Osler was by no means anti-German. Anything but. He liked his German colleagues, and he clearly recognized the paramount position of German medicine in the last decades of the nineteenth century. This opinion appears most articulately in the long mythic description of the travels of Minerva Medica with which he concludes a travel letter published under the title "Vienna After Thirty-four Years":[14]

But this is what happened in all ages. Minerva Medica has never had her chief temples in any one country for more than a generation or two. For a long period at the Renaissance she dwelt in northern Italy, and from all parts of the world men flocked to Padua and to Bologna. Then for some reason of her own she went to Holland, where she set up her chief temple at Leyden with Boerhaave as her high priest. Uncertain for a time, she flitted here with Boerhaave's pupils, van Swieten and de Haen, and could she have come to terms about a temple, she doubtless would have stayed permanently in London, where she found in John Hunter a great high priest. In the first four decades of the nineteenth century she lived in France, where she built a glorious temple to which all flocked. Why she left Paris, who can say? but suddenly she appeared here, and Rokitansky and Skoda rebuilt for her the temple of the new Vienna school, but she did not stay long. She had never settled in northern Germany, for though she loves art and sciences she hates with a deadly hatred philosophy and all philosophical systems applied to her favorite study. Her stately Grecian shrines, her beautiful Alexandrian home, her noble Roman temples, were destroyed by philosophy. Not until she saw in Johannes Müller and Rudolph Virchow true and loyal disciples did she move to Germany, where she stays in spite of the tempting offers from France, from Italy, from England and from Austria.

In an interview most graciously granted to me, as a votary of long standing, she expressed herself very well satisfied with her present home, where she has much honor and is everywhere appreciated. I boldly suggested that it was perhaps time to think of crossing the Atlantic and setting up her temple in the new world for a generation or two. I spoke of the many advantages, of the absence of tradition—here she visibly weakened, as she has suffered so much from this poison—the greater freedom, the enthusiasm, and then I spoke of missionary work. At these words she turned on me sharply and said: "That is not for me. We gods have but one motto—those that honor us we honor. Give me the temples, give me the priests, give me the true worship, the old Hippocratic service of the art and of the science of ministering to man, and I will come. By the eternal law under which we gods live I would have to come. I did not wish to leave Paris, where I was so happy and where I was served so faithfully by Bichat, by Laennec and by Louis"—and tears filled her eyes and her voice trembled with emotion—"but where the worshipers are the most devoted, not, mark you, where they are the most numerous; where the clouds of incense rise highest, there must my chief temple be, and to it from all quarters will the faithful flock. As it was in Greece, in Alexandria, in Rome, in northern Italy, in France, so it is now in Germany, and it *may be* in the new world I long to see." Doubtless she will come, but not till the present crude organization of our medical clinics is changed, not until there is a fuller realization of internal medicine as a science as well as an art.

In this same lengthy letter Osler cites a suggestion which must have had tremendous appeal for him:[14]

At the dinner of the congress His threw out the interesting suggestion (apropos of the presence of Grümbaum and Trevelyan from Leeds, Pratt from Boston, Barr from Portland, Ore., and myself), that the time had come to have an International Congress for Internal Medicine. The physiologists, the laryngologists, the alienist and others have such gatherings, and there now exist in France, Germany and Italy, England and the United States special societies devoted to internal medicine. A congress once in four or five years would be most helpful. We should get to know each other and be able to appreciate better the work done in different countries.

Two years later, in 1910, a Congress on Internal Medicine was held in Wiesbaden, and this may have been the outcome of His's remarks. Osler was unable to attend.

I have mentioned Osler's deep respect for German science, a respect which he extended to their university system in general, commenting that "The universities of Germany are her chief glory, and the greatest boon she can give to us in the New World is to return our young men infected with the spirit of earnestness and with the love of thoroughness which characterize the work done in them."[13] He appreciated the Germanic tradition of professionalism, which he described in a letter to Harvey Cushing:[13]

Now, as you are in part of Teuton, it may interest you to know the general impression one gets of the professional work over here. I should say that the characteristic which stands out in bold relief in German scientific life is the paramount importance of knowledge for its own sake. To know certain things thoroughly and to contribute to an increase in our knowledge of them seems to satisfy the ambition of many of the best minds. The presence in every medical center of a class of men devoted to scientific work gives a totally different aspect to professional aspirations. While with us—and in England—the young man may start with an ardent desire to devote his life to science, he is soon dragged into the mill of practice, and at forty years of age the "guinea stamp" is on all his work. His aspirations and his early years of sacrifice have done him good, but we are the losers and we miss sadly the leaven which such a class would bring into our professional life. We need men like Joseph Leidy and the late John C. Dalton, who, with us yet not of us, can look at problems apart from practice and pecuniary considerations.

Yet I would do Osler a great injustice if I left with you the impression that Germany alone among the European countries interested him. I have already cited portions of two letters from Austria. And he felt a great affinity for France too. In particular, his affection for that country traces to his love of medical history, for he devoted considerable study to the influence of French medicine on medical practice in the New World. And even though Minerva Medica no longer dwelt in Paris, Osler could identify areas where French medicine excelled. "One advantage the French medical student has over all others. To the hospitals of Great Britain and Germany the medical student is admitted as a right; in the United States he is too often only tolerated and not always admitted to the wards! In Paris the hospital is his home."[17]

Speaking of the French people, Osler admired their extraordinary reverence and, identifying himself as "one who believes in the immanence of the mighty dead 'who live again in minds made better by their presence,'" he especially praised their reverence for the great men of the past. He visited Paris on All Saints Day, 1908, and travelled to visit Louis' tomb in the cemetery of Montparnasse. He describes the scene thus:[16]

The main avenue leading to it was an open flower-market, and for three or four hundred yards the cemetery wall was lined with booths for the sale of every sort of emblem and of fresh and dried flowers. Through the "Gates of Grief" a steady stream of people poured, each one bearing some tribute to the memory of a loved one. I stood for several minutes just inside, watching the procession. A group of young schoolgirls passed, each one bearing a bunch of chrysanthemums to lay on the tomb of a fellow pupil or of a loved teacher: close at hand were two Sisters of Mercy arranging wreaths on a vault that looked one of the oldest in the cemetery—perhaps the annual devotion of the guild to a loved member. A little laddie of eight hurried by with a bunch of violets in his hand, running with the ease of one who knew his road. A young mother in deep mourning with a baby in her arms, an aged couple arm in arm, each with a little basket of flowers, two young students, a little old lady with her daughter followed by a footman carrying large wreaths, workmen in rough clothes, soldiers, sailors—a motley group, a touching sight, but on the whole not a sad one. Here and there we could see the stricken heart in the pale set features, but the general impression was one of a cheerful festival, and the glorious sunshine, the bright flowers and the merry voices of the children helped to dispel the gloom of the city of the dead.

Yet there were gloomy events in Paris that winter, events which he observed carefully, and investigated, and then reported with what seems to be great fairness. There is at least a superficially contemporary note to the disturbances at the Paris Medical School on December 21, 1908, disturbances which climaxed an uneasy and at times violent autumn.

Briefly, the events were these. A professional anatomist was imported into the school, replacing the traditional clinician-anatomist. The new professor made a number of changes in the procedure for dissecting which the students found objectionable, and so they objected—sufficiently vigorously so that the dissecting rooms had to be closed for a while. At the same time a change had been made by the examiners who chose, from among the many dozens of clinicians examined each year, those few who would receive appointments as *agregés*,

an associate professorship which was the highest rank to which a Parisian physician could rise on the basis of demonstrated competence alone. This change required the aspirants to take preliminary examinations in anatomy and physiology, subjects with which these men had finished years before.

When the would-be *agregés* protested on the examination day, December 21, they received the support of the sympathetic and already aggrieved medical students. The police were called in. Rioting resulted. The main gate of the school was forced and a crowd of about 250 entered the courtyard.[15] Osler commented, in a letter to the *Times* in London, that "It seems a pity that the police and soldiers were called in." And in another letter he concluded:[16] "A faculty without its troubles is always in a bad way—the waters should be stirred. Some ferment should be brewing; the young men should always be asking for improvements, to which the old men will object. It is a sign of health, and so we may regard these troubles at the Paris medical school—much good will come of them."[11]

The last large group of letters also refer to troubles, but much more serious problems than a short-lived student-police confrontation in Paris. At the end of 1914, Osler began a series of four letters, published in *JAMA* under the title "Medical Notes on England at War."[17-20] And immediately it is evident that he harbored no illusions about what was in store for England. His realism may relate to the certainty he had about the inevitable involvement of his son, Revere, in the war; whatever the reason, Osler quickly saw through the propaganda.

At first blush it really looks as if war were a good thing, a fine tonic to the country at large; but behind all this is the tragedy of the shambles at the front, and the hospitals are full of poor fellows battered and shattered, so that one has not to go far to realize the truth of Sherman's famous words that "War is Hell."[17]

And in another letter he remarks that "It is evidently going to be a 'long, long way to Tipperary' in this war . . ."[18] Osler never needed unusual disaster or tragedy to activate his spirit of compassion, but this emotion was at full flow for those who marched to "Tipperary" and although his prose in these war letters is generally calm and restrained, his feelings show through occasionally. For example, he concludes some remarks on the effects of war on the nervous system by commenting: "The truth is, the trenches have been a veritable hell, and it is not surprising that a good many of the men show signs of severe nervous shock."[18] Equally restrained, but obviously indignant, he spoke of the use of poisonous gases by the Germans: "Certainly the gas is a great addition to the 'frightfulness' of war, but it is to be hoped that the allies may not be forced to adopt such measures of scientific barbarism."[20] Yet I find it interesting Osler did not say the Allies must not use gas—merely that he hoped they would not be forced to do so. In fact, not a particularly forceful denunciation.

This observation leads me to point out what must be obvious, yet is sometimes forgotten by admirers of the great: they are, after all, human. Osler was not a saint, and he was not infallible. And this point can, I believe, be demonstrated from his letters. There may be, for example, a hint of class consciousness and its related callousness in his remarks about an obstetrical ward in Vienna:

Every third day women come to be examined, to see whether their time is at hand. They are arranged on a series of beds, and the assistant takes a student to each case, and examines him on it. No matter how many students are present, all

can have a "finger in the pie," and one feels sorry for the poor women, but Bandl says they don't mind.[3]

I have the same sort of reaction to his description of phosphorus poisoning in Berlin:

Formerly these cases were very numerous, as this was the poison commonly used by the lower classes; now, however, it is out of fashion, because they now know that death by it is neither speedy nor pleasant.[2]

Is this slightly supercilious? If so, certainly the attitude is anything but typical of Osler. But the times were marked by considerable rigidity of class boundaries and distinctions, even here in the United States, all myths to the contrary notwithstanding. So it would be remarkable if Osler was in no way affected by this characteristic of his era.

Before I close, I must mention one additional facet of Osler's humanism. He believed deeply that a special place in history belonged to those rare people we now call "Renaissance men." He admired the polymath intensely. And this admiration invests his remarks about Virchow:

The other morning I could not but feel what a privilege it was again to listen to the principles of thrombosis and embolism expounded by the great master, to whose researches we owe so much of our knowledge on these subjects. At 11 AM each day he gives a lecture on special pathology. Politics and anthropology absorb the greater part of his time. He is a member both of the German Parliament and of the Prussian House of Representatives; and I noticed a day or so ago, in one of the daily papers, an item stating the number of times which each member spoke—I forget in which House—that Virchow had spoken on 38 occasions during the session. It need scarcely be stated that he is an advanced liberal. He is also a member of the City Council—not an idle one either, as the copious literature of the canalization (drainage) system of the city can testify . . . He has been collaborateur with Dr. Schliemann in several of the important works issued on Trojan antiquities. His collection of skulls and skeletons of different races, one of the most important in Europe, will doubtless find an appropriate place in the new Archaeological Museum erected by the Government . . . There are those who grudge him the time which he thus spends on politics and his favorite studies, but surely he has earned a repose from active pathological work . . . and when we consider that, in addition to the classes above mentioned, he is President of the Berlin Medical Society, and edits his *Archiv,* now a large monthly journal, it can scarcely be said that he neglects professional duties.[5]

Virchow was, at this time, elderly, and this observation leads me to comment on an amusing example of apparent inconsistency which crops up in these letters, one which recalls the great controversy in Osler's life. This was the "useless after 40, chloroform after 60" affair upon which I reported at length a few years ago. I shall not recapitulate the story in any detail, but merely say that in 1905 a joking allusion to chloroforming 60-year-olds was blown up by the daily press into a full-scale media-produced event of a kind much more familiar these days. But fifteen years earlier we find Osler saying, in letters published just one month apart, first: "Please note, too, that [Vesalius] was a young man when he published his great work, another illustration of the theory upon which I am always harping, that a man's productive years are in the third and fourth decades."[10] Then, one month later, Osler describes Kolliker, then about seventy, as "a living illustration of the fact that age, after all, is a relative condition."[12]

Other of Osler's theories, beliefs, and campaigns echo through his travel letters. To give a single example, referring in another place to Virchow, he commended an address the great pathologist gave: "His address was most characteristic, and his arguments in favour of vivisection were most appropriate, and will, it is to be hoped, do something to lessen the fanatical

outcry against its legitimate practice, which has disgraced England during the past few years."[4] One of Osler's less well known activities was his vigorous activity combatting the restrictive proposals of the antivivisectionists.

I have spoken at some length about the humanistic attitudes of a man who has been dead more than fifty years. At this point you may fairly say, Osler is a humanist—so what? In my opinion medical education probably, not willfully, is more and more turning out technicians instead of professionals. And the caliber of medical practice will regress as long as this trend continues. The more technical our education becomes, the more we need to have held up before us the example of our forebears. That is what I have tried to do today.

But I have spoken too long, if not by the clock or the program, at least according to Osler's definition. For in one of these letters he stated: "It is a miserable mistake . . . to speak for more than half an hour, but to continue for an hour and a quarter is too much for human endurance . . ."[14]

I thank you for enduring.

REFERENCES

1. Osler, W.: Berlin correspondence. *Can Med Surg J,* 2:231-233, 1873-1874.
2. Osler, W.: Berlin correspondence. *Can Med Surg J,* 2:308-315, 1873-1874.
3. Osler, W.: Allgemeines Krankenhaus. *Can Med Surg J,* 2:451-456, 1873-1874.
4. Osler, W.: The international medical congress. *Can Med Surg J,* 10:121-125, 1881-1882.
5. Osler, W.: Letters from Berlin. *Can Med Surg J, 12:*721-728, 1883-1884.
6. Osler, W.: Letter from Leipzig. *Can Med Surg J, 13:*18-22, 1884-1885.
7. Osler, W.: Notes from the German medical congress—Frerich's festival, etc. *Canadian Practitioner,* 9:184-186, 1884.
8. Osler, W.: Notes of a visit to European medi-

cal centres (editorial). *Arch Med* (NY), *12*:
170-184, 1885.

9. Osler, W.: Letters to my house physicians:
Letter I. *N Y Med J, 52*:81-82, 1890.

10. Osler, W.: Letters to my house physicians:
Letter II. *N Y Med J, 52*:163-164, 1890.

11. Osler, W.: Letters to my house physicians:
Letter III. *N Y Med J, 52*:191-192, 1890.

12. Osler, W.: Letters to my house physicians:
Letter IV. *N Y Med J, 52*:274-275, 1890.

13. Osler, W.: Letters to my house physicians:
Letter V. *N Y Med J, 52*:333-334, 1890.

14. Osler, W.: Vienna after thirty-four years.
JAMA, 50:1523-1525, 1908.

15. Osler, W.: The disturbances at the Paris medical school. The *Times* (London), p. 4,
December 29, 1908.

16. Osler, W.: Impressions of Paris: I. Teachers
and students. *JAMA, 52*:701-703,771-774,
1909.

17. Osler, W.: Medical notes on England at war.
JAMA, 63:2303-2305, 1914.

18. Osler, W.: Medical notes on England at war:
frost-bites and cold-bites. *JAMA, 64*:679-680,
1915.

19. Osler, W.: Medical notes on England at war:
the volunteer army. *JAMA, 64*:1512-1513,
1915.

20. Osler, W.: Medical notes on England at war:
nervous disorders. *JAMA, 64*:2001-2002,
1915.

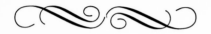

The Relevance of Osler for Today's Humanity-Oriented Medical Student

JAMES A. KNIGHT, M.D.

SIR THOMAS BROWNE has written that "Tis opportune to look back upon old times and contemplate our forefathers."[1] This contemplation is of our renowned fore-bear, Sir William Osler, in company with the medical students of our day instead of his own.

There appears to be much more unrest among medical students today than in preceding decades. The unrest may be related to a number of factors, among them, change and ferment in medical education, recognition of the unavailability of medical services to many groups in our population, changing patterns of delivery of health care, and student involvement in the social problems of mankind.

Medical students are dissatisfied with the education they are receiving. A "dehumanizing experience" is their frequent characterization of how they, as well as patients, are treated.

Not infrequently in the past, students and their physician-teachers focused sharply on the individual patient and neglected the complex social and psychological factors which influence sickness and health. The recent rapid changes in society now prevent such a narrow focus. As a result, students and society are altering their demands on the medical school faster than the school can respond; and both are unhappy with the school.

In seeking to meet the many new demands imposed by society and government, the medical school has neglected students or at least has failed to appreciate today's students with their own set of priorities and concerns. Further, its faculty has not been as open to new knowledge about personal maturation and learning in students as it has been to other new developments.

Probably today's students can best be described as humanity-oriented. What they really want from their teachers and the medical school environment can be identified by asking them. Once the list is compiled, one discovers that Osler's life commitment is profoundly relevant for today's students. Thus, an effort is made in this paper to define the relevance of Osler's educational philosophy for meeting the demands of the modern medical student.

WHAT STUDENTS ARE SEEKING

Ten areas are identified which lend themselves to meaningful interaction between Osler and today's medical students. These areas are described in terms of what students are seeking and how Osler would have responded. The areas are: an educational process relevant to one's goals in life; a sense of priorities; social consciousness; orientation toward the care of the sick and the relief of suffering; community involvement; freedom from bondage to materialism; permission to live today; addictive and contagious passions; recognition of a spiritual dimension to life; and the need for great models.

An Educational Process Relevant to One's Goals in Life

For a number of years Dean Davison has been pleading that medical schools be given back to students.[4] A host of responsibilities seem to take priority over our educational commitment to students. As a result, our students feel that they are second-class citizens in the very institutions which should give them a place of honor and sonship. Their morale is often low and feeds a growing cynicism about the relevance of their educational experience in defining and attaining their goals. They feel a growing alienation from themselves, from one another, and from the patients they serve.

Whenever Osler addressed students, he used the words "fellow students." With such a salutation, a sense of community was formed immediately with those who sought to search with him into the mysteries of health and disease. Brown has expressed well the charismatic and continuing influence of Osler on his students:

> The more we learned, the more wonderful his boundless knowledge seemed; the wider our vision, the more limitless his appeared . . . Because of him our lives have been better, our successes more real, our failures less hard to bear, for through the tangled skein that spells life each of us knows that in him he has, and will always have, a teacher, a friend, and a true fellow student to the end of the chapter.[2]

Osler saw no appreciable interval between the teacher and the taught, only that one was a little more advanced than the other. In such a learning atmosphere, Osler contended that a student would then feel that he had joined a family whose honor was his honor and whose welfare was his own.[12]

Of the many responsibilities of the professor four are absolutely crucial. He has a responsibility first to know and to like his subject; second, to know and to like the learner; third, to know something about and to like learning; and fourth, to know something about and to like teaching. Osler earned a top rating in all four areas.

As a teacher, he had no peer. He spared no effort in preparing himself for his students. Dr. Holman remembers him as "Delightfully informal, erudite beyond comparison, entertaining but surprisingly effective, Sir William Osler enjoyed teaching. So interestingly and compactly were his presentations arranged, it took little effort to remember them."[7]

Osler's love for his students, in fact for all mankind, was never questioned. The phrase from Leigh Hunt's "Abou Ben Adhem" was often used to characterize his life: "Write me as one who loves his fellowmen."

Osler had a deep interest in medical pedagogy and often commented on the ingredients for good teaching and a good teacher. He suggested a school of medical pedagogy in which able young men, aspiring to the position of teachers, could be taught proper methods.[11] Osler's dream of training opportunities for medical pedagogy is only a partial reality today, and medical students continue to suffer from oppressive and stifling methods of teaching.

Osler was imaginative and innovative in his teaching. He made of the hospital a college and did his finest teaching at the bedside of patients. He insisted that the wards be thrown open to students. He assigned his students to the wards and remained there with them. Bedside teaching represented a radically different method of pedagogy to what had been practiced in most medical training centers in the United States up to that time. For example, Dr. Henry M. Thomas, in comparing Osler's teaching methods with what he had seen as a student at the University of Maryland, stated that he had practically no opportunity to get close to patients. Although he had excellent professors, the teaching approach was the old lecture system. He received his medical degree in 1885 without ever having been instructed in physical diagnosis and won a prize in obstetrics without ever having seen a woman in labor.[15]

One of Osler's strongest dislikes was the practice of frequent examinations for students instead of an occasional one. He was convinced that examinations quenched the all-precious investigating spirit of students and made the end and object of study the meeting of certain tests. The examinations were not tests of the capacity to do or to think but how far the student had made himself a phonograph or monotype on which an examiner might play.[11]

The excessive use of the examination remains a part of the student's life in most medical centers and seems to block the development of more effective and personal methods of assessing his progress.

A Sense of Priorities

We dump into the student's lap huge textbooks and smother him with unlimited demands upon his time and energy. Endless classes, assignments, examinations, threats, grading, invidious comparisons, and the treating of knowledge and skill like some salable commodity render the student unable to know what is important, relevant, and meaningful in his educational experience. His teachers should not be astonished when he asks, "Am I in a prison or a kindergarten?"

Osler had the rare ability to place priorities in a proper order. He had such a remarkable sense of what is important and what should be emphasized that many of his judgments have stood the test of time. As Martin Cummings has noted, "With the exception of areas such as clinical therapeutics, which change rapidly, his philosophic and educational views are strengthened rather than weakened by the passage of time."[9]

He encouraged his students in their studies to ask "What do I need to know?" and not "What do you want me to do?" He coveted for the students not the role of a puppet in the hands of others but rather a self-relying and reflecting being. The proliferation of examinations and rigid scheduling of all of the student's time offended Osler's educational sense. We are still struggling to keep faith with Osler's sound judgment on these points but not always with success.

Osler emphasized the blending of the old art of medicine with the new science. In his commitment he had a worthy example in a famous predecessor about whom he often spoke—Herman Boerhaave.[3] When Boerhaave joined the faculty of the medical school in Leyden in 1693, medical practice throughout the world was chaotic and confused by new concepts of chemistry, physics, anatomy, and pathology. Boerhaave organized, distilled, and delivered the useful information from all the rapidly accumulating scientific knowledge of his day and balanced and mixed it with the ancient and traditional art of medicine. Rather than lecture on theory alone, he showed students and his colleagues what to do at the bed-side of sick patients. He selected what was useful from an almost overwhelming mass of discovery and rejected an even greater mass of nonsense which was masquerading as discovery. This unique ability made him *communis Europae praeceptor,* the teacher of the whole of Europe, as a famous student described him.[8]

Osler surpassed Boerhaave in separating sense from nonsense by giving the world a book, *The Principles and Practice of Medicine,* which remained the pattern for text-books of internal medicine for a half century. Both Boerhaave and Osler chose the most illuminating setting available for their teaching—the bedside of the patient.

The information explosion places a heavy burden on the student of organizing and integrating rapidly accumulating scientific knowledge with the ancient and traditional art of medicine. Hopefully the student can gain a perspective from the example of men like Osler and Boerhaave.

Social Consciousness

Students are deeply concerned with the poor and sick who live in the ghetto, the inner city, and isolated rural areas. They want their teachers to share their social concerns and to join them in action programs to correct social and individual ills.

Dr. Gardner recalls one of Osler's clinical lectures to junior students at the Radcliffe Infirmary in which he mentioned "In my behavior to my patients I make no difference whatever between the high and the low, between a duchess and a cook."[6] Gardner comments that in England, at that time, there was a considerable difference between cooks and duchesses and most people were inclined to treat them quite differently. Osler's principle in practice struck the students as excitingly enlightened and humane. His

radiant humanity emerged as a source of extraordinary clinical success.

In Osler's address before medical students at St. Mary's Hospital, London, October 3, 1907, he used the ancient religious term, *calling,* to emphasize what a commitment to medicine entailed:

> . . . You are in this profession as a calling, not as a business; as a calling which exacts from you at every turn self-sacrifice, devotion, love and tenderness to your fellow-men. Once you get down to a purely business level, your influence is gone and the true light of your life is dimmed. You must work in the missionary spirit, with a breadth of charity that raises you far above the petty jealousies of life.[11]

Orientation Toward the Care of the Sick and the Relief of Suffering

The student has as his primary concern the caring for suffering persons. He covets for the patient dignity, privacy and the best of personal care. Osler urged his students never to forget the rights of patients.

Patient after patient that he treated felt the hospital room empty of all except Osler and himself and power. Osler brought insight and a brilliant ability to cope with disease; and then when everything that was human had failed, he brought something less tangible but enduring.

Osler inspired his contemporaries to emulate him in his care of the lowly and downtrodden. In his pity and understanding for those in adversity, his own soul acquired strength.

Patients had absolute confidence in Osler and were certain that there would be no failure from lack of skill or interest in them. To those who had lost courage and hope, he restored the desire to fight. He was a master therapist of the psyche and the soul.

Community Involvement

Town-versus-gown polarizations represent an incomprehensible dichotomy for today's medical student. He craves active involvement in his community's agencies and programs which permit him to practice his humanity. The medical students have begun to break down the walls surrounding our medical training centers and involve themselves in activities beyond the centers' walls.

Over the past several years, with research in the ascendancy and with many full-time faculty members committed only to producing academicians, what Osler dreaded has come to pass: a professorial body remote from its profession and alienated from it. Both students and the public would welcome an Osler to nurture today's embryonic efforts of bringing the community and the medical center into a more productive relationship for health's sake.

Osler had a profound interest in public health and preventive medicine. He stressed the need for a proper and adequate sewerage system and a pure water supply. He played an active role in the control and prevention of illnesses such as typhoid, tuberculosis and malaria.

Because he urged his medical colleagues to participate in the total life and health of the community and set a good example of such participation, he contributed enormously to the welfare of the community through an enlightened profession influencing public opinion in matters pertaining to health, sanitation, and general hygiene.

Much of his profound influence upon the community came through active participation in medical society activities, where he urged regular attendance and greater comradeship for all members of the medical profession. To isolate oneself from the practitioners of medicine in the community because of full-time membership on a medical faculty would have been for Osler a tragic distortion of the physician's calling.

Freedom from Bondage to Materialism

The student is saddened by society's bondage to materialism. It is not that he sees evil in materialism but rather man's failure to use it with grace in the cause of humanity.

Osler seemed to keep himself free from any need to love money for money's sake. One of Osler's students at McGill, Dr. E. J. A. Rogers, in his reminiscences, has stated that Osler's charity reached everyone in whom he could find some measure of sincerity and application. Osler had the greatest contempt for the doctor who made financial gain the first object of his work, and "even seemed to go so far as to think that a man could not make more than a bare living and still be an honest and competent physician."[14] When Osler saw private patients, he conducted his office after the fashion of Dr. James Bovell's—as fast as a fee came in from a well-to-do patient it went out to a poor one. In his lectures to his students he shared the rules which governed his life, one of which was that the poor you have always with you and you must consider them beyond all others. He often quoted Sir Thomas Browne: "No one should approach the temple of science with the soul of a money-changer."

Osler's greatest example in sharing was in the giving of self, and in this example his influence should speak the strongest to our students. In spite of an affluence that blinds periodically, students today are becoming more sensitive to man and to the whole of creation. They are experimenting more and more with going out of their individual selves into the service of others— and their possessions, in whatever form they take, serve with them. Through the bond of sharing, they are integrated into the family of man, unafraid of the grace and the beauty of sharing.

Permission to Live Today

Students beg of their teachers to help them find meaning and joy this moment and this day and abolish the oppressive philosophy of accepting bondage today in order to "live" tomorrow.

Osler, in his student days, became acquainted with Thomas Carlyle's essay "Signs of the Times." A sentence in the essay took him by storm: "Our main business in life is not to see what lies dimly at a distance but to do what clearly lies at hand." The statement became an obsession. He used it as a knight his armor, lived by it, and quoted it often. Into each day he packed the ingredients for the full life, in the finest existential sense. When I see a student totally immersed in some of the oppressive aspects of the medical curriculum and hoping that tomorrow will bring some fresh air, I confront him with the fact that he has for certainty only today and that he should take a moment to read Osler's "A Way of Life."

Addictive and Contagious Passions

Students today usually have some cause or project which they embrace with addictive passion. Emotional and intellectual commitment may be broad and deep, with a touch of madness. They like to see their teachers embrace something with total abandonment. The bland person turns them off as he did the Biblical writer who declared, "So, because you are lukewarm, and neither hot nor cold, I will spew you out of my mouth." (Rev. 3:16)

Osler had two addictive and contagious passions, the fruits of which we enjoy today: his passion for medical history and his love of great books. He blended these two passions and integrated them creatively in his medical vocation.

Osler's love of books led him not only to advise reading and collecting books but also to select special ones as gifts for colleagues, students, and medical libraries. (I get a real thrill when I discover in the Tulane Medical Library on the flyleaf of a rare old volume an inscription from Osler to a medical friend such as John H. Musser.) He gave stimulation and encouragement to individuals, libraries and medical societies to expand and improve their holdings.

He encouraged the study of medical history and biography and found time in the midst of his duties, which might well have availed as an excuse from further intellectual labors, to contribute in large measure to these subjects.

In a dedicatory address given for a new building of the Boston Medical Library, he spoke these memorable words: "To study the phenomena of disease without books is to sail an uncharted sea, while to study books without patients is not to go to sea at all. Only a maker of books can appreciate the labours of others at their true value."[10]

Osler spent a half hour a day reading from the classics and other great writings of the past, including the Bible. His breadth of reading was reflected in his writing and speaking.

He found great models for his passions in both Browne and Burton but especially the latter who swept all known literature into the *Anatomy of Melancholy* and bound it there with what was his own. On every page is the impress of a singularly deep and original genius. On every page quotations abound from all ages and all countries.

Possibly Osler's sense of humor and love of the practical joke may have drawn strength and encouragement from the humor of his great models. It is interesting that Burton, in 1606, wrote a Latin comedy which was acted later at Christ Church,

Oxford. Burton's comedy is a witty exposure of the practices of professors in the art of chicanery. The manners of a fraternity of vagabonds are portrayed with considerable humor and skill, and the lyrical portions of the play are written with a light hand.[5]

In Osler's search through the literature of the past, he sought to offer his students an encounter with their ancestors whose experiences, hopes, achievements and mistakes had made the human condition what it was.

Recognition of a Spiritual Dimension to Life

Osler was a man of faith in an era in which science was in great conflict with religion. Osler and Sigmund Freud were contemporaries. They were heirs of a curious double legacy from the eighteenth and nineteenth centuries, philosophically speaking: eighteenth-century Enlightenment and the reductive naturalism of the nineteenth century. These two traditions came into sharp conflict with the Judeo-Christian tradition, primarily because God was ruled out. Freud embraced the prevailing philosophy of this period as did many other scientists.

Although confronted by this idealogical development and drawing some strengths from it, Osler held to that faith which had served him well from his earliest years—a faith which included the sense that there is a power in the universe that is greater than the individual, that the experience of this power is of supreme value to the individual concerned, and that through this experience life acquires a new meaning, although the experience cannot be arrived at through the operation of reason. While keeping abreast of the times, he held fast to the purpose and ideals embraced in his youth and became identified as a young modern and an ancient saint. He had a splendid model in Sir Thomas Browne who, in his writings such as *Religio Medici,* combined daring skepticism with implicit faith in revelation.

In his school days at Weston, as he sat at the feet of Father William Arthur Johnson, Anglican priest and naturalist, listening to the reading of extracts from Sir Thomas Browne's *Religio Medici* or as he worked with Dr. James Bovell, physician and naturalist, he absorbed some of their qualities. Their qualities lived on in Osler: the gentleness of their hearts toward suffering, their intense curiosity into natural phenomena, and their obsession with the mystical and spiritual.

Today's student, confronted by the increasingly complex ethical issues in research and patient care plus the loss of meaning or sense of alienation in the lives of his patients, would welcome an Osler to help him appreciate the spiritual dimension of man.

Osler's colleagues and students have spoken of his *charisma*. Only when this word is defined correctly does one comprehend Osler's gift of grace: spiritual power and virtue attributed to a person regarded as set apart from the ordinary by reason of a special relationship to that which is considered of ultimate value.

Spiritual power, if truly genuine, has never been associated with evil. One of Osler's biographers, Edith Gittings Reid, may well have given us the real secret of Osler's influence: ". . . to those he cared for on earth he brought life. We will look back and remember that for us was the high privilege of having seen and felt power without evil —a transcendently beautiful life."[13] I wonder if any of our students today will be able to write of their professors that they saw and felt in them *power without evil.*

Osler's students must have seen something of the meaning of love and divinity in Osler's relationship with his wife. An old and intimate friend of Sir Thomas Browne, Reverend John Whitefoot, rector of Heigham, described Browne's wife with the same words with which Lady Osler could be portrayed: ". . . a lady of such symmetrical proportion to her worthy husband, both in the graces of her body and mind, that they seemed to come together by a kind of natural magnetism."[5]

Students are not oblivious to the principle that gives form and meaning to the universe or afraid to recognize the transcendent as that in humanity which keeps going beyond any given situation.

Our students today, as those in Osler's day, will continue to have psychological needs for spiritual direction, for a message of redemptive hope, and a kind of sanction that some things are eternal.

Great Models

Students seek great models after which to fashion their lives. They need to be shown by example how men cope with the vast and impersonal chaos of existence. They need to be exposed to men who make education relevant by integrating compassionate study and informed conduct, by demonstrating a care and concern for what students can become, and by giving students a profound motivation for learning—the hope of becoming better men.

Osler had the remarkable quality of profoundly influencing people both in his personal relationships and through his writings. Osler's biographical and historical addresses have been well described as belonging to the "literature of power," the kind of literature that profoundly influences people in the conduct of their lives.[16]

In assessing Osler's strong hold on young people, many attribute this hold to the perception in his presence of a finer side of life than is commonly seen. His keen sympathy and affection for young people enabled him to enter into their joys and sorrows, and to keep young in defiance of his years. Professor Gulland of Edinburgh captures something of the spirit of Osler in these words:

> In every man he saw, and desired to see, only what was best and so brought out the best in those with whom he had to deal. One left him with the sense of moral uplift and a desire to be more worthy of his confidence and esteem . . . Valuable though his writings are, one would rather have had an hour's talk with Osler than all his books. It was his personality and his personal radiation which gave him the immense power for good which he possessed.[16]

Osler fought for changes in medical education, and many constructive changes of real benefit to students and patients were achieved. His influence was exerted not in argument or controversy but in the force of example. He brought men together through the genius of his friendship and by the way in which he lived his ideals and induced others to share them with him. Our students desperately need such a model today to help them in their professional maturation.

CONCLUSION

Osler's proudest honor was the unwritten title, "The Young Man's Friend." In his writings, care of patients, public addresses, and entertainment in his home, students always occupied a place of honor and royal friendship. At every opportune moment, he touched their lives and lent them grandeur.

REFERENCES

1. Browne, Sir Thomas: *Religio Medici*. London, Cambridge University Press, 1963.
2. Brown, Thomas R.: Osler and the student. In *Sir William Osler, Bart. Brief Tributes to His Personality, Influence and Public Service*. Baltimore, Johns Hopkins Press, 1920.

3. Cushing, Harvey: *The Life of Sir William Osler*. New York, Oxford University Press, 1940.

4. Davison, W. C.: Let's give the medical schools back to the students. *The Pharos of Alpha Omega Alpha, 26*:98-104, 1963.

5. *Dictionary of National Biography*. New York, Oxford University Press, vol. III, pp. 65, 464-468, 1963-1964.

6. Gardner, A. D.: Some recollections of Sir William Osler at Oxford. *JAMA, 210*:2765-2766, 1969.

7. Holman, Emile: Sir William Osler. *JAMA, 210*:2223, 1969.

8. Lindeboom, G. A.: *Herman Boerhaave: The Man and His Work*. New York, Barnes & Noble, 1968.

9. McGovern, John P. and Roland, Charles G., (Eds.): *William Osler: The Continuing Education*. Springfield, Thomas, p. 224, 1969.

10. Osler, William: Books and men. *Boston Med Surg J, 144*:60-61, 1901.

11. Osler, William: The reserves of life. *St. Mary's Hospital Gazette, 13*:95-98, 1907.

12. Osler, William: The student life. In *Aequanimitas with Other Addresses*. Philadelphia, Blakiston Co., p. 400, 1952.

13. Reid, Edith Gittings: *The Great Physician. A Short Life of Sir William Osler*. New York, Oxford University Press, p. 293, 1931.

14. Rogers, E. J. A.: Personal reminiscences of the earlier years of Sir William Osler. *Colorado Medicine*, April, 1920.

15. Thomas, Henry M.: Some memories of the development of the medical school and of Osler's advent. In *Sir William Osler, Bart. Brief Tributes to His Personality, Influence and Public Service*. Baltimore, Johns Hopkins Press, p. 2, 1920.

16. Wood, Casey A. and Garrison, Fielding H.: *A Physician's Anthology of English and American Poetry*. London, Oxford University Press, pp. *viii-ix*, 1920.

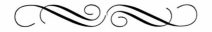
Humanistic Education of The Physician

GEORGE T. HARRELL, M.D.

A REVIEW OF THE PHILOSOPHY of one of the greatest medical teachers, Osler, on the education of students is long overdue. His chief impact was on the clinical years as the students matured into physicians. Osler said he would like to see on his epitaph that he brought students on to the wards to study patients. He believed this act was his greatest contribution to medical education. Osler lived in a time when medicine was being influenced greatly by rapid scientific advances. The studies on bacteria and the development of the entire field of micro- biology established the scientific base for understanding of the major clinical prob- lems of that day, the infectious diseases. The heavy emphasis on science over the last several decades has tended to reduce attention to humanistic values which were the great heritage of medicine in the past. Osler's views and teachings should help us to recognize the importance of these values and keep them in perspective with modern medical educational programs.

TIME OF CHANGE

We live in a time of great change. In the physical world, the industrial revolution has altered patterns of living and affected the diseases with which the physician must cope. The industrial revolution is only a little over two hundred years old and the success in industrial growth began when man learned to harness the natural sources of power. Fossil fuels—coal, oil, and gas— are being used at a prodigal rate, so that it is very likely all of these supplies will have been exhausted in a hundred years or less. Increasingly now, industry is turning to nuclear power which has evolved out of the military development of the atomic bomb, but scientists and engineers are learning to apply the splitting of atoms to peaceful purposes. The supply of uranium for nu- clear power is not unlimited, however. In the future, man must turn to what appears to be an inexhaustible supply of energy, the sun.

The harnessing of power and the develop- ment of machines were made possible by the growth of science. We tend to forget that the sciences we know today as physics and chemistry were developed by physicians in the medieval universities. Most of us are unaware that probably 90 percent of all the scientists who have been trained at the graduate level are still alive today and most of them are still working. The explosion in scientific information is very recent. It is easy to see how humanistic values could be overshadowed and get out of balance with scientific progress.

EVOLUTION OF SOCIETY

Society as we know it today has evolved gradually. Man has been on earth perhaps a million years and organized civilizations have existed for five to ten thousand years. Man has followed the pattern seen in most of the animals. Animals group together in herds for their protection and man has congregated in tribes. This grouping is a basic biologic phenomenon of behavior. We have learned that many biologic studies can be conducted in other species than man with the principles extrapolated to him. The family as a unit appears to have developed when the nomadic tribes learned to cultivate land. With the development of agriculture, man began to settle on his own plot of ground and to reduce his roaming.

The tendency for families to group together led to the development of towns and cities and man became more and more a political person. Towns and cities grew into nations, whose limits were largely determined by geography and economic factors rather than by human behavior. With the improvement of all types of communication and transportation, supranational organizations are evolving so that continents are tending more and more to become the political unit. Civilization is moving gradually toward one world with a very rapid evolution of social and moral values. These values often are changed vastly from what people in some areas have been accustomed to in very recent times.

If we look at medicine in historical perspective, it is apparent that in times past, life was short and perilous. The average life span until the time of the American Revolution was under forty years and only in the past several generations has it begun to approach the biblical three score years and ten. In the past, the causes of disease were unknown. Dramatic epidemics decimated the populations and endemic infections were accepted as part of life, but all disease was shrouded in mystery. Most people died of acute infectious diseases. Until the last two generations, probably more than half of the children ever born in the history of the world died before they reached the age of five years. This fact is still true in underdeveloped and developing countries in all parts of the world today.

Illness was cared for in the home by the family with whoever served as the physician at the time. He may have been a shaman, medicine man, witchdoctor, or later a physician. As far as we know, the first physicians were priests. Certainly, priests were the first educated men. They made observations on natural phenomena about them, particularly celestial events and constructed accurate calendars. With this knowledge, they were able to predict the coming of dramatic events such as eclipses and comets. They surrounded themselves with an aura of magic and miracles, but recorded their observations and passed on their knowledge.

Specialized priests became more interested in people and their diseases than in the physical world, so that physicians gradually grew out of the priesthood. Osler was the son of a minister and the thread of religion as a humanistic study is seen throughout his life.

In the past, the observations on disease made by priests became incorporated into religious laws. Camp epidemics of dysentery were recognized as one of the great scourges of early wars. The Hebrews made this observation and required every soldier to provide himself with a wooden paddle and to emulate the cats in the field. When the soldier had to deposit a stool, he went outside the camp, dug a hole, deposited the excreta, and buried it. This course of action helped to control epidemics of dysentery and the principle has persisted in the pit latrines used today. The scientific reasoning behind the action was unknown. We now recognize that soil microorganisms excrete antibiotics which kill dysentery bacilli, and in this fashion interrupt transmission of the disease. The washing of hands which is part of the communion service in many faiths is a recognition in religious symbolism that the contamination of food by hands is a method of transmitting disease.

In addition to dysentery, other epidemic diseases have affected the course of history. Typhus frequently broke out in military camps and the epidemics may have had more effect on the outcome of battles than the military operations. Zinsser has developed this thesis in his delightful book, particularly in the chapter on the relative unimportance of generals. The Hebrews also observed that when man ate the inadequately cooked meat of swine, he developed muscle pains and often died. Accordingly, the eating of pork was proscribed. We know now that the symptoms were due to trichinosis caused by a parasite which is predominantly found in hogs, but does live in many other animals as well.

In the past, the physician had few effective means of treatment. Often all he could do was to comfort the patient and family and wait for the natural history of the disease to run its course. In the course of his ministrations, he induced faith in himself which in some unexplained way seems to aid the natural process of healing. The physician has always exhibited this faith in

his skills. Indeed, the term "profession" has grown out of this faith in beliefs and the profession or expression of them to others.

The physician had few drugs with which he could work and they were crude natural products. The drugs were usually derived from plants such as the poppy from which comes opium and morphine for the control of pain. Ipecac was found to control some cases of dysentery. It is now recognized that the effective ingredient is emetine which will kill amoebae. Cinchona bark was found to control some cases of recurrent chills and fever, and we now know this action is due to quinine which prevents the growth of malarial parasites. The leaves of oleander when chewed were observed to dilate pupils at the same time the intestinal peristalsis of dysentery was controlled. Women used this observation to make themselves more attractive so that the common name for the effective ingredient became belladonna. As with many drugs when used in excess, the nightshade plant can be deadly.

ROLE WITH PEOPLE

The physician and the priest from whom he originally stemmed always have dealt with people. The interests, motivations and reactions of human beings have comprised the study of humanities. Each individual is different from another. No two look alike, behave alike, and if any physiologic phenomena are measured quantitatively, the data when plotted scatter. If the data on a large enough group are plotted in a linear fashion, a smooth bell-shaped probability curve is found.

People, however, do not wish to be treated from a statistical group approach. Patients want to be handled as individual persons. Individuals are members of a family and in this setting react to the normal stresses of living in an ever increasingly sophisticated civilization. Families live in communities which in turn have personalities that are determined by the cultural backgrounds of the people who comprise the dominant residents. The effects of illness are felt far beyond the patient himself. In addition to the biologic impacts of disease, the social and economic effects are felt on the sociologic unit, the family. All of these effects fall within the field of study of the humanities.

RESPONSIBILITY FOR SERVICE

All professions have a responsibility for service to people. Society grants privileges to a profession and in turn restricts practice to members of it. The profession is expected to maintain its own standards and to develop a code of ethics. Medicine is very proud of its discharge of these responsibilities over the centuries. The practice of medicine involves a highly confidential, interpersonal relationship which requires personal integrity of the highest order. In medicine, this creed originally was set down in the Hippocratic Oath, which we traditionally administer to graduating medical students. The physician serves the patient as an individual and society as a group. The thread of religion in relation to illness is seen in the teaching of the Christian faith that the sick must be helped and not cast out as had been the custom with incurable illness. One of the earlier followers of the Christian religion was Luke, a physician. The same principles are found expressed in one fashion or another in many religions.

CARE OF THE SICK

In the past, the sick were cared for in the home by the family with the help of the physician. The priest, as well, traditionally came to visit the sick. The humanistic thread is seen in the development of hospitals in medieval times as the crusaders returned from the Middle East. The soldiers brought with them leprosy which was easily recognized and dreaded. People had observed that if patients with leprosy were excluded from towns, the transmission of the disease was reduced. The knights hospitalers, when they returned, were quarantined outside of cities. The name hospital became associated with the place where people with infections were isolated to control epidemics. The church as part of its religious teaching accepted care of the indigent homeless sick. The first nurses were probably sisters in the church and this term persists to this day in many countries, even for lay nurses.

The role of improved health as a means of spreading religion is seen in the missionary movement of the past century. Hospitals have been built by various churches to deliver medical care in a religious atmosphere. This trend has been most dramatically publicized in recent times through Schweitzer who had a deep interest in many of the humanities, particularly music and philosophy, as well as in medicine.

Many changes in society which affect the care of the sick have come about as the result of wars. In this country, people live in a period of great mobility. Households now rarely contain more than one generation of a family. In the past, grandparents often lived in the home and helped to take care of the children and the sick. The instruments and machines used in the care of illness have become increasingly complex and expensive. This trend is leading to a centralization of medical care in institutions and a philosophic dilemma has developed. Can one inject an institution into a highly personal relationship such as medical care? Institutionalization makes us face the danger of the loss of the human personal touch in the care of the sick. This danger can be avoided or lessened if particular attention is given to the education of the physician and other health workers.

Changes in the character of illness have occurred in our lifetime. In the past, the chief causes of death were the acute infectious diseases — pneumonia, tuberculosis, dysentery, and malaria. These infections are no longer the chief causes of death. The great killers now are chronic illnesses — heart disease, vascular problems, and cancer. The life span has increased in recent decades and more in women than men. Methods have been developed to interrupt the natural history of disease and to give people a better chance to heal themselves. The prevention of acute infections has been accomplished through control of food and water supplies, immunizations, and later, the development of effective chemotherapeutic drugs.

EFFECT OF SCIENCE

The education of the professions has always been accepted as the role of universities. The original professions were theology, law, teaching, and medicine. Faculties of medicine were a prominent part of medieval universities. The development of the sciences of physics and chemistry by these faculties and their application to improvement in care of the sick introduced the thread of science into medical education. In biology, early scientific studies on genetics were done by Mendel, a monk, through accurate observations on flowers. The scientific principles are now being applied to the study of disease in human beings. The social and behavioral sciences have developed much more recently than the traditional natural sciences. Scientific studies in these fields and the application to medical education are barely beginning.

An explosive growth of knowledge through research has occurred in recent decades, but no amount of research can accomplish change in one phenomenon. The principle of biologic variability must be recognized in education for the health fields. The difference between individuals requires that in the field of medicine, if scientific criteria are to be met, groups of individuals must be studied. In this fashion, individual variations can be smoothed out. A statistical approach can be taken to meet scientific criteria in the conclusions drawn from the studies. When a person becomes ill, however, he wishes to be treated as an individual. An insoluble dilemma is posed. How are data collected on a single individual interpreted against conclusions drawn from studies of a group? The application of data to the individual does not meet recognized scientific criteria. The care of the individual patient is an art, and historically always has been recognized as such. The practice of medicine, however, will remain an art, since it is not in the nature of things, because of biologic variability, that the application of data to the care of the individual patient can be a science.

The art of medicine rests on a scientific base. We apply technical and scientific knowledge to the solution of patient problems. This intellectual process occurs not only in medicine, but in many other professions. An architect sits down with his client, talks with him about his sense of values, his hobbies, how he wishes to lead his life, and what he does with his spare time. The architect then applies his technical knowledge to the solution of the problem and constructs a building which becomes the home. The physician follows the intellectual process of problem solving in his day-to-day work. He sees a succession of people with diagnostic and therapeutic problems.

He must decide if he has enough data to arrive at a conclusion. If not, he plans the collection of data to answer a series of questions in his mind. This process we know clinically as the "work-up."

In planning long-term care of an illness, the physician finds that many of his recommendations are not accepted. The advice is not followed because it conflicts with the cultural background, religious belief, economic resources, and sense of values of the patient and his family. The conflict of religious and other humanistic values with medical recommendations is most clearly seen in child spacing. Nowhere in the world, either in highly developed or developing countries, have the people accepted the known scientifically proven methods for population control. Philosophic, ethical, and religious beliefs also determine the acceptance or rejection of recommendations for prolongation of life in biologically hopeless illnesses.

EDUCATION OF
THE PROFESSIONAL MAN

The preprofessional education of the physician traditionally has been in the liberal arts and classics. In the past, few sciences had been developed on which medicine could be based. In the professional phase of medical education, the humanistic thread should not be lost, and the best preprofessional preparation for the physician is still a broad liberal arts education. With the changing sense of values in society these days, parallel threads of the sciences and humanities should be continued throughout medical education. As a physician, the student commits himself to a never-ending process of self-education. New facts are being accumulated and on them new theories and concepts evolve. Unless the physician commits himself to continuing

life-long education, he becomes hopelessly behind progress in the field.

Physicians should recognize more and more that other humanists can be involved in helping to care for the sick. Many people with mental illness present first to the priest with their symptoms. The priest always has had an adequate education in the classics and humanities, but little in the scientific aspects of behavior and almost none in the biologic aspects of illness. Perhaps these factors need to be examined in the education of the priest, as well as of the physician. If all health science workers are taught together as students, ultimately they should work better together in the community and the health of the people will be improved. When the patient presents a problem to the physician, the doctor will scan the limits of the problem and apply to its solution any discipline, technique, or tool, which he thinks will give him an answer. He is committed philosophically to a multidisciplinary approach to problem solving. As this approach is incorporated into the educational program, the student learns more and more that he cannot depend solely on his own resources as a developing physician. He must utilize technically trained people in various scientific fields as well as helpers from other fields. The priest can be used as a professional colleague to bring his point of view to bear on the design of a long-term program of care which will be accepted by the patient.

ETHICAL AND MORAL PROBLEMS

Many of the major issues in the world today involve not scientific and technical problems, but ethical and moral decisions for which the education of the physician has ill prepared him. An example is the balance between food supply and population growth, which is the largest problem facing the world today. The amount of food grown can be increased by something like a factor of two, or perhaps three, by better use of land, more productive strains of plants, more intensive use of fertilizers, pesticides, and other chemicals. These materials, unfortunately, often upset the ecology. Young people in particular are becoming increasingly concerned with these disturbances of nature, but these practices seem to be the only way in which food supply can be increased.

On the other hand, a great deal of scientific knowledge is available, which will help to control population growth by the use of pills, mechanical devices or surgery. Nowhere in the world has the scientific knowledge available been successfully applied to population control. The reason for lack of acceptance of the available methods is the conflict with the values and beliefs of people. The understanding of these beliefs is the field of the humanities, and the physician must be cognizant of them. Cultural factors in some religious groups in India prevent the reduction of nonhuman use of food. Cattle roam free and are protected even though they may destroy crops and consume food which could be used to feed people.

Abortion is a problem which is now being faced from a legal point of view, and some legislatures are beginning to pass more liberal laws permitting abortion to prevent transmission of inheritable diseases. Many traits are known to be transmitted through genetic mechanisms, but nowhere in the world, with the possible exception of Japan in the last two years, has abortion to interrupt pregnancy for any reason been accepted.

Recent scientific studies have indicated it may be possible to manipulate genes. Artificial insemination, which has proven so effective in upgrading the quality of cattle, is now being used in the human being. A woman can now select the characteristics of the father of her child, if she is fertile and her husband is sterile. Ova have been transplanted in animals. It seems technically possible that a woman who does not ovulate and has not conceived can have an ovum developed by another woman implanted into her fallopian tube where it can be fertilized by her own husband. She can then produce a child. This technique, if required, could eliminate hemophilia as a disease, since it is transmitted through the mother. The moral and ethical problems concerned in these matters have not been fully faced.

Surgical methods have now been developed for the transplantation of normal human organs from a donor to a recipient who needs to have a diseased one replaced. The techniques are further advanced in the transplantation of kidneys than with other organs. Probably fifty to one hundred times as many people who could benefit from kidney transplants are known as is the supply of organs for transplantation. Who will make the decision as to who gets a transplant? The decision is not a medical one, though at the moment, the physician is making it. He is making the decision not on scientific factors, but on ethical and moral grounds. Certain religious groups object even to a blood transfusion. What is the proper philosophic and ethical approach when transfusion will prove life-saving? Does the physician invoke the law and give blood over the religious objections of the family. As scientific advances are made, particularly in the field of tissue typing, these problems will become more and more prominent.

Physicians must face the problem of prolongation of life in medical conditions which are known to be biologically hopeless. Does the physician withdraw all therapy and practice benign neglect or does he take active measures which may relieve a patient from intractable pain and suffering? Physicians are failing fully to recognize human values that have developed through the centuries. In the past, people were born and died in their homes. Now for medical reasons, the mother is taken out of the home to have a child born in the hospital, or to have the patient die there. These dramatic events now occur in an artificial environment away from the members of the family and from familiar possessions and surroundings which the patient has known and loved. Is this practice morally and ethically correct? What effect does it have on the family relationship? These questions are philosophic and not scientific ones, but must be considered and answers found.

What are the moral and ethical bases of human experimentation? Only limited extrapolation to the human being can be made from biologic experiments done in other species. Man inherently is different from the other species and almost no experimental evidence can be extrapolated completely from lower animals to man. Models are lacking in animals for many of the diseases which are seen in man, particularly those which are a result of his adaptation to the environment. The restrictive legislation regularly proposed concerning experiments in animals will hinder scientific attempts to develop disease models of human illness.

Physicians are learning to interrupt the natural history of disease. Scientific measures have been developed to control vectors and reservoirs of infectious diseases. These measures often run into conflict with conservationists, since they may upset the local ecology. Schweitzer applied his reverence for life to such an extreme that even mosquitoes known to be vectors of endemic disease could not be killed in his hospital.

Drugs have been developed which interrupt the natural history of illness. Perhaps the most important drugs are those which alter behavior. It often is forgotten that over half of the hospital beds in this country still are continuously occupied by patients with mental illness. The philosophic and ethical problems arise through the possibility of extending the use of the drugs beyond patients with mental illness to the general public with or without behavioral aberrations. This problem could be a practical one, since one of the major causes of death in all age groups is accidents. Behavior is a large factor in many accidents, particularly in those individuals who are accident prone. Should society require the use of psychopharmacologic drugs to reduce the number of accidents and the cost of caring for the injured which is being borne by everyone?

FUTURE EDUCATIONAL PROGRAMS

How can some of these ideas be incorporated into education programs for the future? The object of medical education is the improvement of individual patient care. The student should study the whole man as a functioning human being, living in a family and subjected to the stresses of living and of his work. The future physician should learn at the very beginning of his professional career that he has committed himself to a continuing process of self-education. He should have discovered in secondary school or college that effective accumulation of knowledge involves individual learning as opposed to teaching by faculty. The educational thread in medicine can be human biology, since the application of the knowledge is to man himself.

Because of the increase in the stresses of living as our society becomes ever more complex and competitive, the study of behavior as a basic biologic phenomenon must assume a greater role in the education of the physician. Many behavioral phenomena, such as sexuality, territoriality, herding, and group behavior, can be taught in lower animals and extrapolated to the human being. Unless the great range of variation in normal human behavior is appreciated, the physician cannot properly interpret the impact of disease on the patient and his reaction to illness. The variation in human behavior with age is readily seen in children, but increasingly as the population ages, the variations in behavior of older people must be recognized. Only after normal variations are recognized can the impact of disease on the patient be evaluated. In the new medical school at Hershey, a Department of Behavioral Science has been developed as a basic science department parallel to physiology and biological chemistry. Behavior is considered a normal physiologic phenomenon basic to all clinical disciplines and not to that concerned with mental illness alone.

The teaching of the humanities in the new school at Hershey is done through a unique Department of Humanities which has educational responsibility in each of the years of the curriculum. The Department is organized with chairs in philosophy and ethics, religion and history of science. The program in the humanities is expected to be a parallel thread to that of the sciences and to have a clear expression, clinically, through patient care in the Department of Family and Community Medicine especially. It is important that the student, early in his educational program, develop his own philosophy and come to peace with himself before he begins to see patients. Only then can he interpret philosophic and ethical problems to his patients and their families

in the community. The role of religion and its effects on the acceptance of the physician's recommendations for care must be better appreciated. A study of religion should encompass those faiths which are found worldwide, since so many people in the field of medicine and in other professional fields come to this country from abroad for a portion of their training.

The educational process must emphasize the role of the family more than in the past, not just in the care of immediate illness, but in the prevention of disease and the delay of complications in chronic illness. The physician should strive toward the maintenance of optimum health in his patient. The recommendations of the physician must relate to the community in which the patient lives and recognize the resources available to the family for the control of the illness anticipated.

At Hershey, a Department of Family and Community Medicine has been developed by bringing practicing physicians from the community with their patients into the medical school. In the first week of the first year, students are assigned families which they follow throughout the four years. The education focuses on the patient in the family setting with the physician bringing in as consultants other people in the community in the field of the humanities, such as the teacher from the school and the priest from the church. A multidisciplinary approach in the broadest sense is made to patient care.

The education of the physician should generate some of the religious zeal for excellence that is seen in other fields. The care of the sick should protect the dignity of the individual patient, and the facilities for his care should be designed from this point of view. The hospital at Hershey has been designed on the acute nursing care floors around all single rooms each with private bath. The emphasis on the family is encouraged through provision of elements of the home on each of the nursing floors. These elements on the hospital floors devoted to specialty medical care remind the physician that even though he may restrict his practice in the future, his recommendations should be made to take into account the impact of the particular disease on the family unit.

Different patterns for delivery of patient care are being explored through the group practice of the Department of Family and Community Medicine. Study is being given to different patterns for financial support of health care. Nationally, great emphasis is being given to prepaid programs which permit the physician to develop a comprehensive, preventive program of care without economically penalizing the patient. As medicine becomes more complex and more instruments, computers and automation are used, the expense of care increases. In addition, the philosophic dilemma is posed of how medical care can become increasingly mechanistically oriented and not lose the compassionate humanistic touch.

The organization of medical care is becoming increasingly institutionalized because of these trends. Can one substitute an institution for an individual physician in the doctor-patient relationship which is essentially a highly personal one? How does the patient react to the efforts to give the physician help by turning history-taking over to a machine or to a less well trained assistant? A computer can analyze a self-administered multiple choice form or the answers given with a light pencil to questions displayed on an oscilloscope tube. Will the patient tell a little black box personal things in his history which he is reluctant to volunteer to the physician face-to-face? Will the patient accept that the information may be available to anyone who has access to the computer and may no longer be confidential? Will the patient accept a computer analysis of the statistical probability of the nature of the illness?

These questions can be subjected to experiment in the next few years. The answers become important since the physician spends a large proportion of his time, regardless of the field to which he restricts his practice, in caring for symptoms of the patient for which he does not find a sufficiently advanced stage of organic disease to explain the magnitude of the complaints. Functional overlay to early organic disease and psychosomatic problems can produce these symptoms. The unraveling of these subtle problems is best done through a careful history taken by an intuitive physician. A computer or other mechanical device cannot recognize or interpret the silent language with which the patient gives the physician hints to things he has on his mind. Humanistic values must not be lost sight of in the education of the physician and indeed all those who are concerned with the delivery of medical care.

Proper recognition of humanism in medicine will lead to renewed dedication of all the health professions to better medical care and improved service to the people. Osler would have approved of this trend.

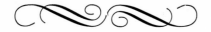

Essay XIII

Humanism in Undergraduate Medical Education*1

DONALD G. BATES, M.D.

Humanism, as a wellspring of conduct toward one's fellow man is more a depth of understanding than a particular content of knowledge. It flourishes best in a personal exchange, in an atmosphere of give and take arising from mutual respect between professor and student, and has as its focus an ever-deepening understanding of one's self. These characteristics of humanism are discussed insofar as they have a bearing on the undergraduate medical curriculum and the way we teach.

"THE TASK AND THE DIGNITY of the human being consist in the individual's willingness to live up to an ideal and to be of help to others." With these words the humanist scholar Ludwig Edelstein defined the teaching of the humanist physician, Sir William Osler. The occasion for these remarks was Edelstein's comments on one of Osler's favourite Hippocratic aphorisms, "Where there is love of man, there is also love of the art." Edelstein went on to make the point that the idea "that medicine itself imposes certain obligations upon the physician, obligations summed up in the magic phrase 'love of humanity,' " appears fairly late in Greek thought. Prior to this, such an obligation to his fellow man was not re-

*From Bates, Donald G.: Humanism in Undergraduate Medical Education. *Can Med Assoc J, 105*:258-261, 1971.

garded as a necessary condition of the physician's craft, though pride in his work was.[2] Perhaps today, at least in practice, we have reverted to something like that earlier view —the love of the art has overshadowed the love of man.

In the 1960's, if not considerably before, the public and profession alike have decried this loss of humanity, and nowhere more frequently than in the literature calling for reform in medical education. But if the goal to be reached has been universally agreed upon, the means for attaining it have not. The following thoughts are addressed to those concerned with the absence of this quality from undergraduate medical education and are an attempt to distinguish some of its characteristics which have a bearing on the curriculum and the way we teach.

Although it is a common practice to call this quality "humanism," that term has many connotations and requires a definition in this particular context.[3] "Humanism" will be used here to refer to an attitude towards other people vaguely described as a "love of man," and will not be employed to mean "humanities studies," however much these may contribute to the skills and knowledge which foster that attitude.[4] This restricted use of the term is employed in the belief that it best expresses the objectives of those who strive for humanism in medical education.[5] The chief concern is to produce physicians who, however great their love of the art, honour the dignity and humanity of their colleagues[6] and patients as fellow human beings.

In undergraduate medical education, humanism thus defined becomes essentially a set of relationships of the student to his teachers, to his subject matter, and, most importantly, to himself. Concerning his relations to his teachers, three factors deserve special mention. First, humanism is a personal thing; it thrives best in a personal setting. The educational milieu must provide opportunities for direct and protracted contact between the individual student and a particular teacher. This is a feature of most graduate study but not of modern professional training, at least in medicine. The development of the elective system, where personal tuition for extended periods of time is more frequent, probably helps. In fact, the kind of relationship made possible between student and professor may be among the greatest benefits of elective programmes. By contrast, formal, mass teaching, designed to instruct on a collective basis, holds out much less hope, whatever the subject matter. It is almost a contradiction in terms to speak of mass indoctrination in a humanism devoted to developing a sensitivity to the liberties, rights, and worth of the individual.

Second, no part of medical education is more crucial for the humanism of the future doctor than his relationship to the teacher during bedside instruction. Yet at no point in the learning process has the love of the art more often overshadowed the love of man. Too frequently a display of clinical mystique or a dazzling performance is enacted with the virtuosity of a prima donna by some teacher who cannot resist the opportunity to parade his mastery of the art before an appreciative, or at least captive, audience. Or, under the guise of humiliating the student into learning, the instructor may resort to corrosive sarcasm and aggressive one-up-manship employed with the malicious enthusiasm of a drill sergeant. Any student who has been crushed with the heavily ironical label of "Doctor" knows the technique well. Such institutional and professional traditions, especially those which might justifiably go under the title of "initiation rites" die hard. But die they must if the student is expected to develop rather than to suppress his sense of humanity. Difficult though it is to arrange, the student's early clinical experience needs to be combined with an exposure to men who have been successful, not only as doctors, but as human beings.[7]

Third, a humanism-fostering relationship is one of interaction rather than of transfer. It does not fit the typical educational model whereby the professor passes on something to the student, suggesting thereby that the former has something which the latter does not. Students are not lacking in this regard. A physician gains in his own humanity through his contact with them. Humanism is not a commodity to be taken or given, but an attitude to be displayed and to be cultivated by a mutual respect between professor and student.

However difficult it may be for a medical school to encourage these kinds of student-teacher relations, the task must be confronted. Without a positive reinforcement of the student's own humanity, and without exemplary models for him to follow, all the courses in the world will not add one inch to his stature as a human being.

This is not to say, however, that the student's relationship to his subject matter is unimportant. If he wants to apply his knowledge with humanity, he must be wise; indeed, he must have that depth of knowledge, that profoundness of understanding which relates learning to the human condition, that is, to the limitations of human understanding and to the varieties of men. From this comes his humanism, his refinement of judgment which uses knowledge with sensitivity as well as accuracy.

What does this imply for medical education? Closely parallel to the need for a protracted personal relationship with an individual teacher is the student's need for an intensive pursuit of a particular subject, whatever that subject might be. Once again medical education compares unfavourably at present with many types of graduate work. Nor is it likely that the medical school can give the kind of depth in understanding which adds a humanistic dimension to one's learning. The unavoidable demands of a professional training involve a broad range of competence and rarely, if ever, permit the establishment of these deeper ties.[8]

But if medical education is, of necessity, deficient in this regard, there is no need to aggravate it with avoidable superficiality. Token courses, given by people with a token knowledge in the humanities, social sciences, or whatever, will not serve the interests of humanism. This is not to say that brief, well-designed courses in these subjects, competently given, cannot enrich a medical curriculum. They can sustain and focus upon medical problems the interest of those already competent in such fields before coming into medicine. They may awaken interests which, if continued voluntarily, will round out the student's education. For the sensitive few, they provide an awareness of just how restricted their medical education is. But even where quality exists, these courses do not serve to infuse a "love of man" into the timetable.

In an effort to develop the human side of our medical students, a good deal of responsibility in recent years has been given to psychiatry and to the behavioural and social sciences. It seems appropriate, therefore, to add a note of caution in this regard.

Much has been said of the dehumanizing effects of science in medicine. But it is not science *per se* which is dehumanizing; it is the application of science to people, the perception of people as objects of scientific study. To the extent that the social and behavioural sciences strive to reduce human behaviour to general laws, they engage in something akin to the scientific enterprise. In the twentieth century, these sciences, particularly psychology and psychiatry, have attempted to add behaviour, mental performance, and attitudes to the domain of scientifically explained phenomena. Considerable explanatory power, with encouraging signs of practical application, has arisen out of this approach. But, as has just been pointed out, it is contradictory in a fundamental way to approach people's problems scientifically and humanely at the same time. In the disciplines in question, dehumanizing is deliberate and essential. But unfortunately this means that, instead of the witness' testimony being regarded as an accurate record of his bodily or mental experience, the testimony becomes a part of the phenomena which are to be studied objectively. They are seen as only the superficial manifestations of deeper processes of which the patient is unaware and which only the trained professional understands. The possibility must be entertained that, ironically, the very disciplines being counted on in undergraduate medical education to create an understanding of man's behaviour and a compassionate treatment of him may be contributing to making the physician cold and calculating. Understanding, in a scientific sense, does not guarantee empathy; on the contrary, it can lead to precisely the opposite.[9]

Humanism in medical education cannot

be isolated as a subject, but must be woven into the fabric of the student's experience, particularly into his relationships with his teachers and with his subject matter. It must also permeate his understanding of himself. The wellspring of humanism is self-knowledge.[10]

In concentrating on the student's understanding of how other people react to situations, our medical schools risk neglecting his deeper insight into his own behaviour. Objectifying patients is easily picked up as a technique and is powerfully effective as a defensive mechanism for the physician. He can put his patient down, assert his authority over him, and mould the patient's problem into terms and categories with which the physician is familiar. Only with difficulty and considerable maturity does he learn to "play fair," using the same rules to understand his own behaviour toward the patient that he uses to interpret the patient to himself. All of the student's biological and a good deal of his psychological training is with reference to the person-out-there. Very little attention is given to the me-in-here.

During the course of his undergraduate education, the student must discover much about himself as a person, and as a professional, in terms of his interactions with his patients and colleagues. His ultimate responsibility is to serve. It is the medical school's task to cultivate whatever natural inclinations he has for a life of service.[11] Professional traditions, medicine's increasingly esoteric nature, its therapeutic successes, and society's adulation all pull toward giving the impressionable student the sense that he is becoming a master rather than a servant. But professional arrogance, the prima donna, and the virtuoso are the most serious threats to humanism in medicine. Without wishing to sound cynical, I would like to suggest that self-knowledge, a truly deep in-

tellectual honesty about oneself and where one most rightfully fits in society, invariably leads to humility. The love of man is obscured neither by the love of the art nor by the love of self.[12]

In summary, humanism, as a wellspring of conduct toward one's fellow man is more a depth of understanding than a particular content of knowledge. It flourishes best in a personal exchange, in an atmosphere of give-and-take arising from mutual respect between professor and student, and has as its focus an ever-deepening understanding of one's self. Much of what has been specified as necessary to the cultivation of this humanism in undergraduate medical education is idealistic. But then, humanism in the physician is an ideal. If a sufficient portion of a medical faculty shares this ideal, it will be realized. For one conviction shared by those who exemplify humanism is that "the task and the dignity of the human being consist in the individual's willingness to live up to an ideal," as well as "to be of help to others."

REFERENCES

1. Some of the thoughts in this paper were first incorporated in an unpublished report to the Dean of Medicine, McGill University, by a committee charged with examining the objective of undergraduate medical education. The report was entitled "Undergraduate Medical Education and the Needs of Society." Subsequently, some of these ideas were expressed in "The Future of Humanism in Medicine,'" a panel discussion within the symposium "Humanism in Medicine, as portrayed by the life of Sir William Osler," Galveston, Texas, April 21st and 22nd, 1970.
2. Ludwig Edelstein: The professional ethics of the Greek physician. In Temkin, O. and Temkin, C. Lilian (Eds.): *Ancient Medicine*. Baltimore, The Johns Hopkins Press, pp. 319-

384, 1967. Edelstein had given the original version of this paper as The William Osler Lecture in the History of Medicine, Faculty of Medicine, McGill University, December 9, 1955. Osler had discussed this Hippocratic aphorism in his essay *The Old Humanities and the New Science,* an address before the Classical Association, Oxford, May 16, 1919, London, J. Murray, 1919.

3. For a history of the connotations of "humanism," see Allen, P. S.: The humanities. *Proceedings of the Classical Association of London, 14*:123-133, 1917.

4. According to Allen, *(ibid.* p. 127f.), in the usage of late antiquity, "humanitas" was commonly equated with "philanthropia," a kind of general benevolence to all mankind. This was contrary to the practice of Cicero who used the term to refer to the learning of a gentle man, a free man, viz. the liberal arts. See Rand, E. K.: The humanism of Cicero. *Procedings of the American Philosophical Society, 71*:207-216, esp. p. 210f, 1932. For a discussion of the meaning of "philanthropia" in antiquity, see Edelstein, *op. cit.*

5. A separate paper is being prepared on the role of the humanities in undergraduate medical education.

6. By this is meant all those engaged in helping people with problems. That there is an especially great need for the physician to have a proper perspective of his own profession and a sensitive awareness of others is now commonplace in the current literature on medical education.

7. "Upon the life, not the lips, of the master is the character of the boy moulded," Sir William Osler: Intensive work in science at the public schools in relation to the medical curriculum. In *The School World,* p. 15, 1916.

8. See Ennio C. Rossi: Why is the medical profession estimable in the individual but not in the generality? *Perspectives in Biology and Medicine, 8*:230-240, 1964-65. Rossi concludes that "the best place for students to learn human values in medicine is in the research laboratory." In arriving at this apparently paradoxical conclusion, Rossi seems to have observed the humanistic benefits which flow from such studies without having entertained the possibility that it is the depth of them and the relative intimacy of the learning environment rather than the orientation and content of the studies themselves which are the determining factors. Altogether, I do not find his delineation of "human values" and "social values," as applied to physicians, persuasive.

9. I refer here, of course, to the physician with an undergraduate and basic internship acquaintance with these subjects, not to fully-trained psychologists and psychiatrists who have learned to apply their generalizations to themselves as well as to their patients.

10. Cicero repeatedly spoke with approval of the Delphic utterance, "Know Thyself," (Rand, *op. cit.,* p. 213). See also Ludwig Edelstein: Andreas Vesalius, the humanist. In *Ancient Medicine,* p. 453, ftn. 39, where he discusses this maxim.

11. Osler's admonition, "let us remember that we are the teachers not the servants of our patients," (The treatment of disease. *The Canada Lancet, 42*:899-912, 1908-09) seems to contradict this. Osler was speaking of the need to prevent the subservience of professional judgment to the desire to please the patient, and, in that context, his advice is acceptable. Still, Osler's manner of expression perhaps betrays a concept of the profession which is now becoming dated.

12. To Cicero, self-knowledge leads to an appreciation of the divine in oneself. To the Renaissance mind, Man is the measure of all things. But, in our post-Darwinian, post-Freudian world, when men have fallen even from Man's Grace, humility seems the most likely outcome of knowledgeable introspection.